Hynes.

WHAT EVERY WOMAN SHOULD KNOW ABOUT BREAST CANCER

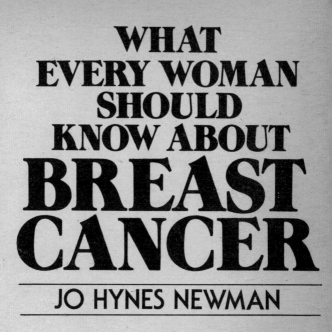

JO HYNES NEWMAN

MAJOR BOOKS • CANOGA PARK, CALIFORNIA

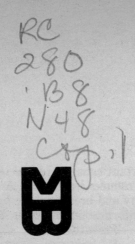

Illustrations by Bonnie Holmes-Johnson

MAJOR BOOKS
21335 Roscoe Boulevard
Canoga Park, California 91304

PRINTED IN THE UNITED STATES OF AMERICA

ISBN 0-89041-082-8

Library of Congress Catalog Card Number: 76-8656

TABLE OF CONTENTS

relationship with your doctor, as equals, so you won't hesitate to ask him your unanswered questions.

Before I let go, I'd like to thank my friends who helped me through this project: Yvonne MacManus, my editor, originated the idea for this book; her determination to create a breast cancer handbook that everyone can understand was a driving force behind this book. Barbara Cox, of Belles-Lettres literary agency, ably handled all the business details between writer and publisher. My very special thanks go to my dear friend Sherry Halperin who was responsible for involving me in the project at the beginning.

Denys Hutchinson, Assistant Service Director for the Orange County Unit of the American Cancer Society, was most helpful in providing information about the Reach to Recovery Program and manufacturers of breast forms. I am very grateful for her assistance.

I cannot begin to give enough thanks to Hazel and Bill Tezak who, during the long months of writing this book, not only cared for my sixteen-month-old son, Steven, but also loved him as they would their own grandchild. Their free-flowing love for Steven enabled both mother and son to move successfully through a very important period in both our lives.

And, most of all, I thank my husband Bob for his help and encouragement. In the late hours when I was too tired to think straight, Bob would carefully read over the manuscript and pick out points that needed further clarification and those that were overdone. His friendly suggestions and medical expertise added greatly to the finished work.

J.H.N.
July 1976

Introduction

Breast cancer. How often have you seen those terrifying words emblazoned across the pages of women's magazines? *Betty Ford, Happy Rockefeller, Marvella Bayh.* Imagine your own name in their place. Too painful to think about, right?

If you think that breast cancer can't happen to you, you're wrong. One out of fifteen women is destined to have breast cancer. That statistic seems so cold and impersonal that it's easy to disregard its significance. Think of it this way: every seventeen minutes, around the clock, three new cases of breast cancer are diagnosed. And every year, more women die of breast cancer than American soldiers were killed in ten years of the Vietnam War.

If you can still feel complacent about missing your annual checkup, then you are denying reality. *Breast cancer could happen to you.*

"Is there nothing I can do to protect myself?" women ask. Yes, there *is* something you can do: you can help to protect yourself through your own vigilance and self-education. Through this book, you will learn the early warning signs of breast cancer. Every effort has been made to keep this guidebook simple and easy to understand. Naturally, there are some medical terms; but if you don't know what they mean, there is a Glossary at the back of the book that explains their meanings.

You don't have to understand complex physiology to have a basic understanding of the cancer process. Cancers or tumors are, very simply, groups of cells whose growth rate has gotten out of hand— cancer cells reproduce themselves at lightning speed. As the number of cancer cells increases, they naturally take up more and more space. Gradually, normal cells are displaced, and the affected organ ceases to function normally.

When the cancer completely takes over its original site, it starts looking for more room to grow. Some cancer cells are sent out as scouts, so to speak. These scout cells migrate into the lymphatic system via the lymph nodes.

The lymphatic system is like a connecting network throughout the body. Within the system there are lymph nodes; these nodes act as purifiers, filtering out larger bacteria and viruses. Once inside the bloodstream, lymph is treated just as any other body waste and is eventually excreted through the urine.

Normally, the lymph nodes filter out bacteria and viruses that would otherwise get into the lymph channels and spread disease throughout the body. Sometimes, cancer cells successfully pass through the lymph nodes and into the channels. Once inside the lymph channels, cancer cells can travel throughout the body and set up new tumor sites, or what doctors call *metastases.*

You might think of this process as a form of guerrilla warfare: first, cancer cells set up a central command post, which we call "the primary tumor." Then cancer cells break through the body's defenses (the lymph nodes) and proceed to set up other bases of operation (metastases). Most of this operation is carried out in total secrecy; there is usually no pain until the cancer is already well established.

What causes the initial cancer formation? Researchers all over the world are working to answer that question. Some cancers are probably caused by external agents such as cigarette smoke, industrial pollution, or radiation; some may be caused by viruses; still others are related to hormone imbalances. Someday, when the causes of cancer are clearly understood, you will probably read books on preventing breast cancer. But for now, the best we can do is to be alert to the possibility of breast cancer: *if breast cancer is caught in its earliest stages, it* can *be cured.*

Most people associate the word "cancer" with an inevitably slow and painful death. Actually, this is not normally the case. Remember that cancer is a most insidious disease: it proceeds stealthily toward its goal of destruction, causing almost no pain until its most advanced stages. Once the painful stage is reached, the end may be very near. That's why regular self-examination and annual checkups are so important to catch cancer in the early stages.

Early discovery, followed by prompt surgery, usually results in a cure. Depending on the type of cancers they had (and there are too many types to list), 85 to 100% of women whose breast cancers had not invaded the lymph nodes are still alive five years after undergoing surgery. Even when their lymph nodes are already cancerous at the time surgery is performed, 45 to 50% of breast cancer patients are still living five years later. And most of these women are still alive ten years after their surgery.

Have you ever wondered why some people get breast cancer and others don't? Cancer doesn't choose its victims quite as arbitrarily as you might think. For example, women get breast cancer ninety-nine times as often as men do. Women over the age of thirty run a far greater risk than do their younger counterparts. Women who live in the northeastern United States are more likely to get breast cancer than are their more southern sisters. The ages at which women begin to menstruate and have babies are other factors. There is even evidence that women with certain personality traits are particularly prone to breast cancer. This book includes a checklist to help you determine whether you are a "high risk" for breast cancer. Just remember that no one is immune to the disease, so we must all be wary; women in the high-risk group must be extra cautious.

Monthly self-examination, using the technique described in this book—coupled with annual examination by a physician—greatly increases the chances that even if you do get breast cancer, it will be caught early enough to be treated and cured. Some women, thinking they wouldn't recognize a lump if there was one, hesitate to examine their own breasts. The first time you try it, it does seem a bit strange, but with practice you will come to know your breasts so well that even a slight change is very noticeable. You will even have a slight edge over your doctor, who can't possibly remember the exact shape of your breasts from year to year.

Those of you who haven't been to your doctor lately will be pleasantly surprised. Recent medical advances make it possible for specialists to diagnose breast cancers before there is even a discernible lump. These examinations—called mammography, xeroradiography, and thermography—are quick and usually painless. You'll learn all about them in this book.

Despite improved technology, a biopsy or tissue sample may be required to make the final diagnosis. Before undergoing such a procedure, the patient must sign a very confusing document that is commonly known as the "consent for surgery." More than a few women have awakened after a biopsy expecting to find only a small incision and found instead the massive bandages covering a radical mastectomy. Together we'll sort through this assortment of medical and legal terms to understand exactly what the consent form means. You *can* avoid the unpleasantness of the unexpected and the fear of the unknown.

One of the most important things you can do for yourself is to find a doctor you can trust and with whom you can develop a good doctor-patient relationship. If you were planning to go into partnership with someone you'd certainly take the time to investigate all the details of the transaction, wouldn't you? It just doesn't make sense to entrust your life and the health of your body to someone you don't know anything about. In this book you'll learn how to check out a doctor's credentials and how to tell if you can successfully relate to each other.

It is an unfortunate fact of life that, no matter how vigilant we are about our monthly self-examinations and annual checkups, some of us will get breast cancer. Those who do develop the disease should understand the basics of the treatment we face. Do you know the difference between a simple mastectomy and a radical mastectomy? Or between a partial mastectomy and a lumpectomy? Do you know why some surgeons refuse to perform anything less than the radical procedure? Do you know why you may have to have radiation treatments, hormone therapy, or chemotherapy? You will have the answers to these questions when you've finished reading this book.

The most terrifying thing about hospitalization and surgery is not knowing what to expect. We'll go over every detail of your stay in the hospital, from day of admission to day of discharge. You'll know exactly what will happen before, during, and after your operation. You'll learn what medicines you'll be taking and what exercises you'll be doing during your convalescence. Your cooperation in these treatments is vital to your recovery.

There is one complication that cannot be treated with medicines and exercises: breast cancer surgery is almost always accompanied by temporary psychological disturbances. Of course the degree of disturbance varies widely, but fears of rejection, disfigurement, and social isolation are always present. After all, the breast is symbolic of a woman's sexuality as well as of motherhood. In a society that is so breast conscious, loss of a breast seems an unthinkable horror to most women.

How can we deal with these fears? Some women simply turn inward and brood, forever mourning their fate. Other women spend hours in the beauty shop to make themselves feel more attractive. But most of us have too many other responsibilities to spend much time brooding, and few of us can afford the luxury of frequent visits to the beauty shop. This book gives a more rational approach to dealing with post-mastectomy depression—that is, a process through which the mastectomized woman can identify her real self as separate from her body. Does that sound terribly deep and psychological? It's really only common sense. Try this little test: list five assets which enable you to function successfully in relationships with your friends and family. I'll bet that your breasts didn't make the list! Assets such as friendliness, ability to forgive, or willingness to help a friend are far more important, and they're not at all dependent upon the shape of your body. Your real self actually *is* separate from your body, regardless of what Hollywood and Madison Avenue would lead you to believe.

Even if you never have breast cancer, the chances are very great that a friend or relative will have the disease. You can aid their recovery by helping them to alter their own self-concepts, away from the "body beautiful" image and toward the "beautiful person" concept. Specific suggestions for ways you can help are covered later in this book.

But we're getting ahead of ourselves. You probably have more questions now than you did when you started reading! That's terrific! We learn by asking questions, so *let's keep asking!* What is breast cancer like? How will it affect my life? How can we overcome the problems that come with the cure?

Now, instead of relying on third-hand horror stories from well-meaning friends or overly technical explanations in medical books, you will finally get straight answers to your questions about breast cancer. Ask questions as you read this book. Ask questions of your doctor, the American Cancer Society, the National Cancer Institute.

Ignorance and fear are breast cancer's greatest allies. Education and vigilance are its greatest foes. You have a very powerful weapon against breast cancer within yourself—your own determination to fight that unacceptable one-in-fifteen chance.

Chapter One

WHO GETS BREAST CANCER?

By analyzing the detailed medical histories of women who have breast cancer, scientists have discovered that some women are much more likely to get breast cancer than are other women. These susceptible women are called the "high risk" group. You can determine for yourself if you are a member of this group by completing the following questionnaire.

For each question, check the answer or answers that apply to you. When you have answered all the questions, turn to page 21 to analyze your answers.

1. My sex is:
   _____ A. Male
   _____ B. Female / .

2. My age is:
   _____ A. Under 30 years /
   _____ B. 30-40 years
   _____ C. Over 40 years ⌐

3. My marital status is:
   _____ A. Single (never been married)
   _____ B. Divorced
   _____ C. Married /

4. I have had____?____full-term pregnancies:
   _____ A. None
   _____ B. Two or less
   _____ C. Three or more /

5. My first full-term pregnancy occurred at age:
   _____ A. 18 years or younger
   _____ B. 19-34 years /
   _____ C. 35 years or older
   _____ D. I have not had a full-term pregnancy

6. I began to menstruate at age:
   _____ A. 12 years or younger
   _____ B. 12-15 years
   _____ C. 16 years or older /

7. My ovaries were removed surgically:

_____ A. Before age 35 years

_____ B. Between ages 35-50 years

_____ C. After age 50 years

_____ D. My ovaries have not been /
removed

8. I have menstruated:

_____ A. Less than 30 years /

_____ B. More than 30 years

9. My height is:

_____ A. Shorter than average

_____ B. Average /

_____ C. Taller than average

10. My weight is:

_____ A. Lighter than average

_____ B. Average /

_____ C. Heavier than average

11. I have lived most of my life in:

_____ A. The United States

_____ B. A Scandinavian country

_____ C. The British Isles

_____ D. Israel

_____ E. A country not named above /

12. The town or city where I live is:

_____ A. An urban center

_____ B. A rural area /

13. I live in:

_____ A. The San Francisco Bay area

_____ B. The northeastern United States
_____ C. Neither A nor B

14. My race is:
_____ A. Caucasian /
_____ B. Black
_____ C. Other

15. My socio-economic status is:
_____ A. Lower class
_____ B. Lower middle-class /
_____ C. Middle-class
_____ D. Upper middle-class
_____ E. Upper class

16. My religion is:
_____ A. Christian
_____ B. Jewish
_____ C. Other /

17. My diet includes:
_____ A. No meat
_____ B. Some meat /
_____ C. Lots of meat

18. I have had benign breast disease (non-cancerous disease such as mastitis or cysts)
_____ A. Yes
_____ B. No /

19. The following members of my family have had breast cancer:

_____ A. My mother
_____ B. My sister
_____ C. No one in my family has had it /

20. I breast fed my babies:
_____ A. Yes /
_____ B. No

21. My ear wax tends to be:
_____ A. Wet and sticky
_____ B. Dry and flaky /

22. I have had my uterus removed (hysterectomy) but my ovaries were not removed:
_____ A. Before age 45 years
_____ B. At age 45 years or later
_____ C. I have not had a hysterectomy /

23. I have taken birth control pills:
_____ A. Before having any children
_____ B. After the birth of my first child
_____ C. I have not taken birth control /
        pills

24. I regularly take the drug reserpine for treatment of high blood pressure (hypertension):
_____ A. Yes
_____ B. No /

25. My breasts are:
_____ A. Small /
_____ B. Average
_____ C. Large

ANSWERS

1. *If you answered B, circle your answer.*
   Females are ninety-nine times as likely to get breast cancer as men. Men who take estrogens—as therapy for cancer of the prostate, for example—are much more likely to develop breast cancer than are other men.

2. *If your answer was B, circle your answer. If you answer C, circle your answer and draw a big checkmark in the left margin.*
   Women over the age of thirty-five are much more likely to get breast cancer than are younger women. Seventy-five percent (75%) of all breast cancer victims are over age forty.

3. *If your answer was A, circle your answer.*
   Women who have never married are statistically about two and one-half times as likely as married or divorced women to get breast cancer.

4. *If you answered A or B, circle your answer.*
   Women who have given birth to two or fewer children run twice the risk of women with three or more children.

5. *If you answered C, circle your answer. If you an-*

swered A, draw a big plus in the left margin.

Women who have had one or more full-term pregnancies before the age of eighteen seem to have some sort of lasting protection against breast cancer. Oddly enough, women who have their first full-term pregnancy after the age of thirty-five run a greater risk of developing breast cancer than do women who were never pregnant at all.

6. *If your answer was A, circle your answer.*

The earlier a girl begins menstruating, the more likely it is she will develop breast cancer.

7. *If you answered A, give yourself a great big plus in the left margin. If you answered B, give yourself a small plus.*

Women whose ovaries are removed surgically before the age of thirty-five have a 70% effective protection against ever developing breast cancer. Women having this surgery between the ages of thirty-five and fifty gain some protection too.

8. *If you answered B, circle your answer.*

Women who menstruate thirty years or more are about one and one-half times as likely to get breast cancer as are women who menstruate less than thirty years.

9-10. *If you are age fifty or older, and you answered C for both these questions, circle your answers.*

In the fifty years and older age group, the majority of women with breast cancer are taller and heavier than average.

11. *If you answered A, B, C, or D, circle your answer.*
Women who live in these countries are more likely to develop breast cancer than are women who live in other countries.

12. *If your answer was A, circle your answer.*
Women living in urban areas are more likely to get breast cancer than are women in rural areas.

13. *If you answered A or B, circle your answer.*
The San Francisco Bay area and the northeastern United States (especially the New York-New Jersey areas) have the highest incidence of breast cancer.

14. *If your answer was A, circle your answer.*
Caucasian women run the highest risk. Unfortunately, black women who do get breast cancer generally do not fare as well as white women, even when they receive exactly the same treatment.

15. *If you answered D or E, circle your answer.*
Women in the upper-income brackets develop breast cancer more often than do poorer women.

16. *If you answered B, circle your answer.*
Jewish women are more susceptible to breast

cancer than are other women. However, Jewish women seldom get cancer of the cervix.

17. *If your answer was C, circle your answer.*

High fat consumption correlates with a greater risk of developing breast cancer. In the Orient—where diets contain little meat, and most frying is done with soya oil—the incidence of breast cancer and colon cancer is very low.

18. *If you answered A, circle your answer.*

Women with histories of benign breast disease (and especially those who have taken birth control pills for six years or more) are more likely to get breast cancer.

19. *If you answered either A or B, circle your answer and draw a checkmark in the left margin. However, if you answered both A and B, draw five checkmarks in the margin.*

A woman whose mother or sister had breast cancer runs two to three times the normal risk of developing the disease. If both her mother and sister had breast cancer, her risk is fifteen times the norm. If any of the relatives had bilateral breast cancers (cancer in both breasts) the risk is increased by a factor of six-to-nine times the normal.

20. *You don't get circles, checks, or pluses on this question.*

For some time scientists believed that breast feeding gave lasting protection against breast cancer. Modern studies indicate that there is absolutely no relationship between breast feeding and breast cancer. The woman who breast feeds her children is just as likely to get breast cancer as the woman who bottle feeds her babies.

21. *If you answered A, circle your answer.*

Most women who get breast cancer have the wet and sticky kind of ear wax. This isn't quite as far-out as it seems; the kind of ear wax you have is inherited, and so is the tendency toward breast cancer.

22. *If your answer was B, circle your answer.*

Surgical removal of the uterus without simultaneous removal of the ovaries increases the risk of breast cancer when the surgery is performed at age forty-five or later.

23. *If you answered A, circle your answer.*

Women who took birth control pills before the birth of their first child are three times as likely to get breast cancer as are women who did not.

24. *If your answer was A, circle your answer.*

Recent studies indicate an association between reserpine use and breast cancer. If you are presently taking reserpine, do not stop taking it without consulting your physician first. You must keep taking it until you can get an alternate prescription for control of your high blood pressure.

25. *You don't get circles, checks, or pluses on this question, either.*

Women with big breasts do not get cancer any more often than do women with small breasts. However, by the time their lump is discovered, the chances are that the big-breasted woman's tumor is more advanced, simply because of the difficulty of feeling a very small lump in such a breast. Therefore, the small-breasted woman has a statistically greater chance of *surviving* breast cancer.

SCORING

This test cannot tell you whether or not you will get breast cancer. It can only indicate whether you run a relatively high risk or a low risk for the disease. Figure your risk in this way:

1. *Each circled answer increases your risk.*
2. *Each checkmark increases your risk greatly.*
3. *Each plus decreases your risk greatly.*

Starting with the average risk of one-in-fifteen, you can calculate your own risk to be slightly greater if you have several circled answers and no pluses. Your risk is substantially greater than one-in-fifteen if you have numerous circled answers or if you have any checks. On the other hand, if you scored any pluses, your risk is quite a bit less than one-in-fifteen. However, no one is immune to breast cancer; a plus doesn't "guarantee" that you'll *never* have the disease. All women should practice monthly self-examination and have a checkup every year. Women who are high risks should see their doctors more often.

Chapter Two

WHAT CAUSES BREAST CANCER?

If personality, socioeconomic status, and religion sound a little farfetched as indicators of breast cancer risk, then read on. There are logical, scientific explanations for all these indicators. This may be difficult reading for those who have never studied science, but you can gain some understanding of this complex issue by skimming the text rapidly, not stopping to follow the medical logic closely. For those of you who are interested in the "whys" of breast cancer, the details and logic of modern research studies should provide interesting reading.

It is difficult for most laymen to understand why

progress in cancer research is so slow—that is until they see just how difficult it is to pin down the specifics of breast cancer. The plain fact is that medical science cannot yet identify any *one* cause of breast cancer. Many factors seem to interact to cause and promote breast cancer growth.

The Virus Theory

Viruses are disease-causing agents which are so tiny that they can't even be seen with an ordinary microscope. In fact, viruses weren't even discovered until modern times with the invention of the electron light microscope.

Viruslike particles have been found inside breast tumors and also in the breast milk of women suffering from breast cancer. The same particles can also be found in the breast milk of many normal women, but in far fewer numbers. The number of breast milk-virus particles is much greater in normal women with a family history of breast cancer than in normal women with no history of the disease in their families.

The evidence sounds impressive, but it is only circumstantial. Cancer cells, whether immature (not yet evident) or advanced (clinically evident) could merely harbor the viruses and not be caused by them. The relationship is not yet clear.

If these viruses do cause breast cancer, then how are the viruses, and hence the disease, transmitted from one person to another? In mice, the virus can be transmitted through breast feeding, but in humans that is not very likely. Among the many mother-daughter cases of breast cancer there is no higher incidence of breast feeding than among the normal population. Many daughters of women with breast cancer were bottle fed only and yet they developed the disease.

Another possible route of transmission is through the sperm and egg. In rats this has been documented, and it is very probably the case in humans as well. Some family histories show that breast cancer can be transmitted through the father. Several other kinds of viruses have been found in human sperm and eggs, so why not breast cancer viruses?

The Hormone Dependence Theory

Research studies have proven that some breast cancers depend on the presence of certain hormones for their growth. The suspect hormones include the estrogens, the adrenal steroids, and the thyroid hormones. Never mind the strange-sounding names of these body chemicals; the theory of hormone dependence is really amazingly simple.

Estrogens: Estrogens are more commonly known as the "female" hormones, though they are normally found in both males and females. In premenopausal women, the estrogens, produced by the ovaries, are responsible for initiating and maintaining the menstrual cycle. They may also be responsible for initiating and maintaining some breast cancers.

Basically there are three types of estrogens in a woman's body: estriol, estradiol, and estrone. The latter two are the strongest estrogens and have the greatest carcinogenic (cancer-causing) effect. Estriol, however, not only has *no* carcinogenic potential, but it also seems to act antagonistically toward the estradiol and estrone, thus negating their cancer-producing potential.

During pregnancy, when the amount of all three estrogens is increased dramatically, the ratio of the "good" estrogen (estriol) to the "bad" estrogens (estradiol and estrone) rises to ten times greater than normal. The protective effect of early pregnancy (specifically, before age eighteen) indicates that the most important period for the initiation of breast cancer cells is the decade after the onset of menstruation. Evidently the great amount of estriol in the body during pregnancy can effectively kill, or at least permanently suppress, immature cancer cells. Once breast cancer is more firmly established, the effects of estriol on cancer cells are less noticeable.

The amount of estriol produced can be determined by a urine test. Asian women, who very seldom develop breast cancer, have very little estriol in their urine; this means that they metabolize or utilize the hormone very efficiently, leaving little of it to waste. On the other hand, women with breast cancer utilize the two "bad" estrogens more efficiently than do normal women. This lends weighty evidence to the hormone-dependence theory.

Strangely enough, estrogens may be the real culprits in women who consume great amounts of fats in their diets. You see, bacteria which are normally present in the large intestine have the ability to mix up dietary fats and biliary hormones to make more estrogens. The resulting surplus of estrogens could encourage growth of breast cancers.

Millions of young women are currently consuming excess estrogens in the form of birth control pills. Unfortunately, we do not yet know what the long-range effects of this practice will be in regard to breast cancer. Most human carcinogens have an incubation period of about ten years; that is, the cancer does not become evident until at least ten years after exposure to the cancer-causing substance. Since birth control pills have been widely available for only about twelve years, it is still too early to judge the possible effects.

We do know, however, that since 1963 (just about the time that birth control pills really became popular), there has been a steady increase in breast cancer among women. Recent studies show that women who used the pill before the birth of their first child are three times as likely to develop breast cancer as are women who did not take the pill before having children. Women with a history of benign breast disease who take the pill six years or longer are also more susceptible to breast cancer. The pill may not be the cause of these women's cancers, but further investigation is imperative.

But estrogens are not the only culprits in the development of breast cancer. Statistics show two peaks of breast cancer incidence: one at around 45-50 years of age and one at 65-70 years of age. The younger age group are still influenced by estrogens.

But the older women, long past menopause, are probably affected by an imbalance of adrenal steroids.

Adrenal steroids: These are hormones produced by the adrenal glands, located on top of each kidney. Women with breast cancer have a very low level of adrenal steroids in their urine, which means that these women metabolize the hormones very efficiently. The apparently normal sisters of women who have breast cancer also have a low level of adrenal steroids in their urine. We know that these women are likely victims of breast cancer themselves. Someday a simple urine test for the presence of adrenal steroids in the urine may be used to predict breast cancer risk.

In postmenopausal women the adrenal steroids are the main source of estrogens (through biochemical transformation). The women with breast cancer, and their sisters who metabolize adrenal steroids so well, are making a much greater than normal supply of estrogens. We already know that an oversupply of estrogens is conducive to breast cancer growth.

Thyroid hormones: It has long been observed that women with a history of hypothyroidism (insufficient production of thyroid hormones) fare better than normal women when they both get breast cancer. This fact holds true even when the cancer is diagnosed very late, at a very advanced stage. The explanation of this phenomenon lies in the relationship between thyroid function and the "good" estrogen, estriol. You see, the greater the amount of thyroid hormones in the blood, the less estriol is produced. This causes the ratio of "good" estrogen to "bad" to swing over in favor of the "bad," and thus breast cancer growth is promoted. The fewer thyroid hormones produced, the higher the ratio of "good" estrogens to "bad"; in this way, breast cancer growth is discouraged by hypothyroidism.

The Immunologic Theory

The immune response is the body's natural defense against invasion by disease-causing agents. The body is programmed to recognize body intruders by their unique protein coating (the antigen). When an intruder's presence is sensed, antibodies are sent out to the site of invasion to neutralize the invaders by combining with their antigen. Somehow this combination of antigen and antibody is more easily "eaten up" by white blood cells than is the antigen alone. This is the immune response—the process responsible for the "tissue rejection" that you heard so much about when heart transplants were in vogue.

The immune response is usually quite effective in dealing with a limited amount of tumor antigen. For example, the immune response can keep cancer cells dormant for many years and thus maintain a clinically disease-free state. Women with breast cancer often have cancer cells escape into their bloodstreams, but the immune response usually takes care of these cells in short order. It is when the primary or original tumor is very large that the immune response ceases to be effective against it.

When a woman has advanced breast cancer that has spread to other parts of her body, her immune system is overwhelmed by the presence of so much tumor antigen. But when the primary tumor (the breast cancer) is removed, the immune response may recover enough to fight off, or at least control, the growth of the metastases. The significance of this phenomenon for the choice of mastectomy technique is discussed in Chapter Nine.

Paradoxically, there are problems when the immune response is overstimulated, too. Hormones may play a large part in these problems. The adrenal steroids have a suppressive effect on the immune response. Estrogens, on the other hand, can stimulate the immune response to the point that it becomes self-defeating. In this case, an excess of antibody is produced. The oversupply of antibody then combines with the tumor antigen in such a way that the white blood cells cannot "eat up" the resulting combination. The antigen-antibody complex actually serves as a protective coating for the tumor!

The interplay of immunologic and hormonal influences on breast cancer growth is clearly demonstrated in women who suffer from a disease called myasthenia gravis, or MG. MG patients have a very low level of adrenal steriods in their urine; as we know, this means that they metabolize or utilize the hormones very efficiently. It also happens that malignancies are exceedingly common among these women and that 40% of those malignancies are breast cancers. When the thymus gland—a gland largely responsible for immune function—is removed from a woman with MG, her chances for developing breast cancer drop to the normal one-in-fifteen; simultaneously, the level of adrenal steroids in her urine increases to the normal level.

The Genetic Theory

Evidence of a genetic link in the development of breast cancer is indisputable: when one identical twin gets breast cancer, her sister usually gets it too—in the same breast, in exactly the same spot. The predominance of mother-daughter cases, and even paternal grandmother-granddaughter cases, indicate a genetic causation in some women. That there is a very high incidence of breast cancer among men with Klinefelter's syndrome (a genetic disease) is further evidence.

Again, hormones are probably linked to heredity. In order for a woman's body to produce estrogens from the raw materials available, certain chemicals called enzymes must be present. There is no question that the presence or absence of these enzymes is inherited. Excessive production of estrogens, and consequent breast cancer growth, can run in families.

The tendency to have wet and sticky ear wax is also inherited. As we mentioned in Chapter One, most women with breast cancer have the wet and sticky type of ear wax. The fact is that both the breasts and the glands that manufacture ear wax are similar in microscopic structure; the process by which ear wax is produced is biochemically similar to that by which breast milk is made. Under these circumstances, it doesn't seem too far-fetched to assume some sort of genetic control over breast function as well. Analysis of ear wax may someday prove to be means of predicting who is and is not likely to get breast cancer!

Defects in fat metabolism, also a factor in breast cancer growth, may also be discovered through ear wax analysis someday. The wet and sticky type of ear wax is found very frequently among patients with a disease called arteriosclerosis, or fatty deposits in the arteries. Consumption of great quantities of dietary fats greatly aggravates this condition as well as encourages growth of breast cancers. If the defect could be discovered early in life, dietary precautions might help prevent both breast cancer and arteriosclerosis.

Other Theories

Many women believe that a hard blow to the breast can cause breast cancer. There is absolutely no reliable scientific evidence that injury to the breast causes breast cancer. A history of injury preceding the discovery of a breast cancer is not too remarkable. Just think how many times you've bumped your breasts on the sharp corner of a cabinet door or had a breast pinched hard by a toddler climbing over your shoulder! Everybody injures their breasts at one time or another.

A link between breast cancer and environmental agents has been established in animal experiments. Scientists have bred a special strain of mice in which 100% of the animals spontaneously develop breast cancers—that is, they develop tumors for seemingly no reason at all. When some of these newborn mice were flown from the United States to a laboratory in Australia, the incidence of breast cancers in these mice dropped to almost zero! But when their normal food and sawdust bedding were flown in from the U.S., their breast cancer rate again approached 100%. Obviously the breast cancers were caused by a combination of environmental carcinogens (in the food and bedding) and some inherited defect in the mice.

The evidence in humans is not nearly as conclusive. Statistics show that countries with the highest breast cancer rates are also the countries where the most solid fuel, coffee, and tea are consumed. There may or may not be a connection here, but the statistics point out areas that need further study.

Nitrites, chemicals commonly used to preserve meats like bacon and hot dogs and some cheeses, are proved carcinogens in rats; humans metabolize nitrites exactly the same way that rats do, so the substances may very well cause breast cancer in humans, too. Nitrites are also found in many vegetables (most notably spinach) and in some drinking water, tobacco smoke, and pesticides. Regulation of our diets and our environment may turn out to be necessary for controlling breast cancer.

Certain drugs also appear to cause or promote breast cancer growth. Reserpine, a drug used to treat high blood pressure, may very well cause breast cancers, but we do not yet know this conclusively or how. Other drugs, such as some tranquilizers and antidepressants, promote cancer growth by raising the level of prolactin in the blood. (Prolactin is a hormone normally secreted during pregnancy to stimulate milk production.) In rats, prolactin has been proven carcinogenic; in humans, the role of prolactin is poorly understood. Normal nonpregnant women have little or no prolactin in their blood. Pregnant women do have high levels of prolactin, but the beneficial effects of estriol, the "good" estrogen, seem to outweigh the bad effects of prolactin. It is possible that nonpregnant women, without the benefit of an increased estriol level, may be setting themselves up as future victims of breast cancer by taking these drugs over a long period of time. Certainly these women should be carefully watched by their physicians.

Broad spectrum antibiotics, used indiscriminately, could represent a hazard too. These drugs work by suppressing the immune response; this could logically promote cancer growth. The present practice of using broad spectrum antibiotics over many years to treat young girls with acne should be examined closely, especially since we know that the teenage years are the crucial years in breast cancer development.

A very rare influence in the development of breast cancers is massive irradiation. Women exposed to atomic bomb blasts have a very high incidence of malignancies. In the past, when high-voltage fluoroscopy equipment was used for frequent placement of chest tubes in tuberculosis patients, breast cancers sometimes resulted. Today's X-ray equipment is low voltage and, when properly used, *does not* cause breast cancer.

High socioeconomic status probably increases breast cancer risk only because it generally correlates with later marriage, fewer children, and higher dietary fat consumption. The roles of these factors have already been discussed.

The relationship between personality and breast cancer is most interesting. Experiments, in which mice were made neurotic by submitting them to intermittent electric shocks, showed that psychological stress does indeed correlate with increased breast cancer risk. When a woman is under stress, her adrenal glands secrete more adrenal steroids than they normally would. As we have already learned, the adrenal steroids suppress the normal immune response and thus promote cancer growth. In addition, psychological stress activates fat metabolism, which in turn promotes cancer growth by adding to the body's supply of estrogens.

How nice it would be if scientists could identify some single cause of breast cancer! But the chances of that happening seem almost nonexistent. So far, the evidence points to an extremely complicated interaction of viral, hormonal, immunologic, and genetic factors that are further influenced by the environment. Someday, perhaps, we'll understand just how all these factors work together to cause breast cancer.

stress in a constructive manner can very well influence her chances of getting breast cancer.

Let's look at the psychological history of Sally T., a mythical conglomerate of many women. Sally is the perfect example of the breast cancer personality:

Sally T. was the third child in a family of six children; two of her siblings, one brother and one sister, died in early infancy. When Sally was only nine years old, her mother died—Sally never quite forgave her mother for dying. The little girl took over feeding and caring for the younger children after her mother's death. On the surface, she was the perfect mother substitute, loving and self-sacrificing; inside, Sally hated giving up her childhood to take over motherly duties.

When she began to menstruate, Sally's reaction was one of disgust and shame. She had received no explanation of the facts of life from her mother, and no one bothered to explain things now. Sally's father, anxious to keep her at home, repeatedly warned the now teenaged Sally to "stay away from men." Other relatives interspersed their praises of Sally's domestic prowess with tales of the other young girls her age who were busy with dating and parties. "Tramps, that's what they are!" Sally's aunt would say. Since she herself would have loved to go to parties and meet boys, Sally soon learned to think of herself as a tramp. To punish herself, she continued to suppress her normal social and sexual urges.

When the younger children grew up and no longer needed Sally's constant attention, she finally married. In keeping with her self-concept of "tramp," Sally married Jack, an alcoholic. Sally seems sure that she can help Jack overcome his drinking problem; she scrimps and saves so that they can get along on the few dollars Jack manages to earn at odd jobs. Really, Sally has absolutely no intention of reforming Jack, since she subconsciously believes that her life of hard work and no luxuries is her punishment for resenting her mother's death.

Jack hardly ever wants to make love, since most of the time he is too drunk to perform. This is just fine with Sally; she has never had an orgasm and finds sexual intercourse distasteful. Sally was very surprised when she became pregnant, although she had taken few precautions to prevent it. Now that the child has reached toddler age, Sally hovers over him constantly, worrying and watching, playing at the role of "mother" once again.

When Sally is angry at Jack or their child, she always manages to swallow her anger. She forces herself to smile and be pleasant. In fact, the other women in her neighborhood admire her calmness; they are totally unaware of the anger that rages inside their friend.

Do you recognize any of yourself in Sally? Admittedly, her faults are exaggerated. But she does exhibit those personality traits that, in their more subtle forms, are found widely among breast cancer victims. Let's look at each of these personality traits more closely:

1. *She is a middle child in a large family.*
   Breast cancer patients are almost never only children.

2. *One or more of her brothers or sisters died at birth or early in infancy.*

3. *One of her parents died when she was a child.*
   This left her with an extraordinary amount of responsibility within the home.

4. *She has an unresolved conflict with her mother.*
   Sally never forgave her mother for dying. But sometimes when it is the father who has died, the conflict centers on the mother's having taken over the dead father's role.

5. *She received little or no sex education.*
   Except for such warnings as "All men want to do is use you," she was completely unprepared

for the onset of menstruation; she reacts almost hysterically with shame, fear, and disgust. She suppresses her normal sexual desires. As a wife, she is nonorgasmic and repulsed by sex.

6. *Her marriage is stable, but unhappy.*

She marries a man who will make no demands on her, sexually or otherwise. Usually he is an alcoholic or unable to hold down a steady job for some other reason. At the same time, she carefully complies with his every whim—she is masochistic in this regard.

7. *She is overprotective of her children.*

She probably didn't want any in the first place. It is almost as if she wishes that one of the terrible things she imagines could occur, would really happen, and relieve her of her responsibilities.

8. *She is unable to express hostility.*

She prefers, instead, to hide behind a facade of pleasantness.

How can a woman's personality influence her chances of developing breast cancer? Somehow, sustained stress has a depressive effect on the body's natural defenses and thus encourages cancer growth. (This subject is covered in detail in Chapter Two, "What Causes Breast Cancer?")

Studies have shown that the women who survive longest after mastectomy are those who openly express their anger and hostility. On the other hand, most of the women who do not survive for long after their surgery are women who are passive by nature—women who do not confront those who have hurt them or express their hostile feelings. It seems that a woman who spends a lot of energy keeping up a false front of pleasantness has too little energy left over to fight off the cancer.

If there is interaction between mind and body, then it should work in reverse as well. Does it? There is one documented case of tumor shrinkage after intensive psychotherapy—without chemical, hormonal, radiation, or surgical intervention. This is just one case, however, and it doesn't necessarily prove anything. There were no laboratory tests done to monitor the patient's normal defenses. It is possible that some undetected change in his immune response was responsible for the tumor shrinkage.

Biofeedback, the science of mind control over bodily functions, offers more evidence. One doctor has his patients concentrate three times daily on curing their cancers; they visualize armies of white blood cells attacking and destroying their tumors. The daily meditations have spectacular effects on the patients' responses to radiation treatments.

Interaction of mind and body is as yet not completely understood. But there's no denying that it exists and that it is strong enough to influence not only who gets breast cancer, but also, who survives breast cancer. With this in mind, the importance of maintaining a healthy emotional outlook is obvious. So, if you see any of yourself in Sally T., you must count it just as you would a circled answer on the previous questionnaire. If you can't handle stress, your risk of developing breast cancer is definitely higher than one-in-fifteen.

Chapter Four

HOW DO I EXAMINE MY BREASTS?

More than 90% of all breast cancers are detected by the women themselves. Of course, some of these discoveries are entirely accidental; a husband or lover discovers a lump during foreplay, or the woman feels a lump as she rubs on body lotion.

Self-examination refers to the deliberate examination of her breasts by the informed woman. We all know how important early detection of breast cancer is—yet many women never examine their breasts. "If there's anything there, I don't want to know about it!" they claim; as if their ignoring a lump would somehow, miraculously, make it go away. Other women, influenced by erroneous information about sexuality, equate touching their breasts with masturbation, and consider it wrong or sinful.

Let's set the record straight right now. Self-examination of the breasts can in no way be considered masturbation. Indeed, the breasts are erogenous zones. So are the lips and the ears. But you apply lipstick and wear earrings, don't you? The method of breast self-examination you'll be learning in this book will not arouse you sexually, if you are concerned about that.

Now—on with the method. First you should know that self-examination is not suitable for everyone. It works best for women with small- to medium-size breasts which are soft in texture. Women with large or very firm breasts will have more difficulty identifying a lump. Therefore, if your breasts are large and/or firm, be extra conscientious about your annual checkup since you can easily miss a tumor in your own examinations.

The best time to examine your breasts is in the middle of your menstrual cycle, two weeks after your period begins. Immediately before, during, and after your period, slight lumps or swellings are common and mean absolutely nothing. So if you wait until the second week of your cycle, you can avoid confusing these harmless lumps for tumors.

It is most convenient to begin the breast self-examination while bathing. When the skin is wet and slick it is much easier to examine the breasts without undue rubbing.

Begin by examining your right breast. Put your right hand behind your head, as shown in the picture. Now imagine that your breast is a clock face, with invisible numbers; twelve is at the top of your breast, three is to your left, six at the bottom, and nine to your right.

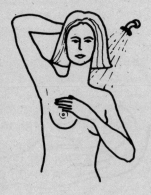

Place the fingers of your left hand at twelve o'clock. You should use only the flat surfaces of your fingers, and never the tips. Holding your fingers in place, gently push the breast tissue around in a small circle. (The movement of your hand must come from the elbow and shoulder; if you bend your fingers or wrist, you're doing it wrong.) As you make the circular movement, try to distinguish any lumps or bumps under the skin.

When you have finished making the circle at

twelve o'clock, move on to one o'clock. Continue around each of the twelve "invisible numbers." Then move your fingers inward about an inch, and go around the clock face again, as shown in the illustration.

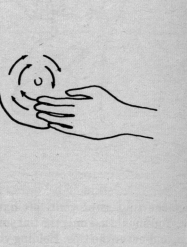

Finally, make an additional small circle over the areola (the dark skin surrounding the nipple). Squeeze the nipple *gently* between her thumb and forefinger to check for discharge.

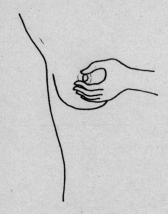

Repeat the entire process on your left breast. This time, put your left hand behind your head, and use the fingers of your right hand to perform the examination.

It's a good idea to do this examination twice—once sitting up (as in the shower or bathtub), and once lying down on your bed. Lie on your back and put a small pillow under your shoulder on the side you're examining, as shown in the illustration. Put that hand behind your head, just as you did in the previous examination. Now make your small circular motions to check for lumps and bumps under the skin. In this position, your breasts are flattened against your chest wall (your ribs and the muscles which cover them), so they may feel slightly different and reveal more. Otherwise the examination is exactly the same.

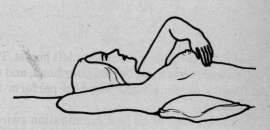

Once a month, before you dress in the morning or when you're drying off after a bath, stand in front of a mirror and look at your breasts, as you hold both hands above your head. Check to see that your breasts look exactly as they always have. If your breasts always looked the same size and suddenly one is larger than the other, call your doctor. If the skin around your nipples becomes puckered (like an orange peel, for example), you'll want your doctor to examine your breasts, And, if your nipple turns inward when it used to stick out, an examination by a physician is in order.

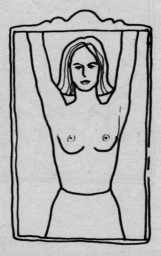

Next, rest your hands on your hips and again compare your breasts. Very few women have truly symmetrical breasts, so don't worry if your breasts are slightly different in size or hang unevenly— provided that is their normal appearance. Your only cause for concern is a *change* from what is *normal* for you.

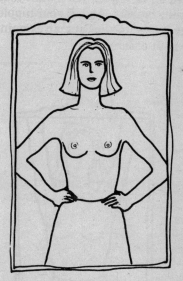

If you examine your breasts regularly, you'll come to know them so well that even a very slight change is readily apparent.

Chapter Five

WHAT IF I FIND A LUMP?

If you should find a lump during your self-examination, *don't panic!* Several other, completely harmless, diseases can cause symptoms just like those of cancer.

One of the most common of these diseases is fibrocystic disease. (Don't confuse fibrocystic disease with cystic fibrosis—they're two entirely different things!) Fibrocystic disease is absolutely harmless, and almost all women will have it at some time in their lives. It is most common in women thirty to forty years old. During the menstrual period, the lumps of fibrocystic disease can be very painful, but they are not cancerous.

A fibroadenoma can also mimic breast cancer. These solid lumps are very common in the breasts of teenage girls and young women in their twenties. The lumps are totally harmless.

Other harmless conditions that simulate breast cancer are papilloma (nipple discharge), hematoma (a lump under a bruise, usually resulting from an injury to the breast), and mastitis (a breast infection characterized by swelling, pain, and lumps). It is even possible to have eczema on the nipples. This benign skin condition causes the areola to pucker and look rather odd.

The point of describing these harmless conditions is *not* to provide you with a ready store of excuses for avoiding your doctor. There is absolutely no way you can tell whether your lump, nipple discharge, or whatever, means breast cancer or something else. *Only* your doctor can tell the difference, so see him!

Don't delude yourself by thinking that breast cancer only happens to someone else. It can very well happen to you. Avoiding a physical examination could be the equivalent of signing your own death warrant. At the same time, rushing out to put your will in order and then sitting back waiting to die is hardly a rational approach either. If your lump is benign, your inaction amounts to sentencing yourself to years of unnecessary anguish. Be smart. See your doctor and find out what is happening inside your body.

There are probably several thousand women reading this book who have already discovered a lump and have done nothing about it. Are you one of them? It's so easy to think up an excuse, but very few excuses stand up to the light of logic and scrutiny. Is your excuse one of these?

1. *"It's just a little lump, so I don't think it could be anything really serious."*

   There is absolutely no correlation between tumor size and the degree of malignancy. In fact, the most malignant tumors cause the earliest symptoms. A small lump could be (1) a very malignant tumor at a very early stage, (2) a not-so-malignant tumor at a more advanced stage, or (3) one of the harmless conditions mentioned earlier. Do you really want to take a chance?

2. *"I've had so many cysts. I'm sure this is just another one."*

   Women with a history of benign breast disease—and that includes cysts—have a greater than average chance of developing breast cancer. With that fact in mind, it is ridiculous to forego a physical examination with an excuse like this one.

3. *"But it doesn't hurt!"*

   Cancer usually doesn't hurt until it has reached a very advanced state. By the time it starts hurting, it could be too late.

4. *"I've never been sick a day in my life!"*

   So what? There's always a first time. If this is breast cancer, it could be the last time, too, if you continue to ignore it.

5. *"My breasts always feel lumpy. It's just normal for me."*

Many women do have lumpy breasts. For them, self-examination may be useless. These women must see their doctors regularly for diagnostic testing (see Chapter Seven). Only a doctor, with the aid of thermograms, mammograms, xerograms, and possibly tissue samples, can make the diagnosis.

6. *"My father had cancer and they couldn't do anything for him."*

Breast cancer is one kind of cancer that doctors can do something about. Breast cancer can be aggressively and successfully treated. If you sit around making excuses, though, it may be too late by the time you see your doctor. Call him today.

7. *"I can't afford to take the time off from work. I've got three kids to support!"*

If you tell your employer the importance of your visit to the doctor, you may be able to get the time off without losing any pay. Even if you do have to lose some pay, it's still worth it. Isn't it better for your kids to do without something temporarily than to do without you entirely? That's exactly what may happen if you continue to ignore the warning signs.

8. *"I would be too embarrassed."*

It is impossible for a doctor to examine a patient's breast when she's wearing her clothes. So if you are too embarrassed to be examined by a male doctor, then find a woman doctor. There are enough women doctors around today for you to find at least one in or near your community. The next chapter will tell you how to go about finding a new doctor.

9. *"I'm afraid of doctors (or hospitals or operations)."*

Which are you more afraid of—cancer or doctors? You can take steps to assure yourself of your doctor's competence, and you can find out how good his hospital is in advance. You'll learn how in the next chapter.

Now that you're no longer hiding behind a lot of excuses, you can make an appointment to see your doctor. If you don't already have a doctor, you can get one—even if you have no money to pay one. Keep reading and you'll find out just how to go about the awesome job of doctor-hunting.

Most women find a gynecologist by asking for recommendations from their friends. While your friend can tell you if her own doctor is a likable person, she cannot tell you whether he is professionally competent. Only another physician, observing that doctor in action, can judge his professional competence. Your friend's doctor could be a social master but a medical disaster.

If you're lucky enough to live near a medical school, finding a good doctor should be no problem. Simply call the school, or get a copy of their catalog from your local library, to obtain a list of their clinical faculty. These are doctors practicing within the community, who also assist in teaching medical students. They are preselected for their medical expertise and teaching skills, so you have a readymade list of doctors who can give you expert medical care and who should be able to explain things to you clearly. If these men or women are too busy to take on any new patients, they can at least refer you to someone else whose medical skills they respect.

If you don't live near a medical school, the search for a good gynecologist becomes somewhat more complicated. But whatever you do, don't use the yellow pages of your telephone book as your "physician selector." *Anyone* can list himself there with absolutely no proof of his qualifications.

A much better way to find a doctor is to look at the *Directory of Medical Specialists* at your public library. All the doctors included in this book are board certified in their specialties—they have completed several years of specialty training (the residency) after graduating from medical school, and they have passed extensive tests (the boards) of their knowledge.

To use the directory, look first under the section devoted to diplomats of the American College of Obstetrics and Gynecology; these are doctors who specialize in the diseases that are unique to women. In this section, look in the subsection that most accurately describes the city in which you live. For example, if you live in Houston, Texas, you'll look under Texas—Houston. In this way, you narrow down your list of qualified gynecologists to those who practice in or near your own city.

By reading these doctors' qualifications, you can learn a great deal about them. You learn when he was born (and therefore his age), and when he graduated from medical school (which gives you some idea of his experience). The date he passed his board examinations is also included, as are the hospitals he admits his patients to, and any teaching or research positions he holds. In general, if a doctor has completed an approved residency, passed his boards, and practices in a hospital with a good reputation, he is probably a careful and thorough physician. If he's part of a group practice (several doctors who work together), that's even better; his partners have already screened him carefully since they know that his reputation affects their own.

If you don't have access to the directory, you can call your county medical society for their recommendations. Usually they will give you at least three names so that you have a choice. But remember that a recommendation from the medical society does not necessarily mean that these doctors are better than others. It means only that the doctor recommended has asked the medical society secretary to give out his name so that he can acquire new patients. If you use this method to find a doctor, be sure to ask for his credentials before committing yourself to his care.

If you cannot afford to go to a private doctor, you have several alternatives for medical care. Your city or county, or possibly a charitable organization, may run a free clinic near your home. These clinics are designed to provide free and low-cost health care to anyone who needs it. Usually they are staffed with young doctors who volunteer their services in order to gain experience while still a resident. (A "resident" is a doctor who has graduated from medical school and is currently doing his specialty training before taking the boards.) Your county health department should have information on free clinics in your area.

To treat patients who are not sick enough to hospitalize, most county hospitals have outpatient departments that provide low-cost medical care to those who qualify. Visiting an outpatient department is very much like going to a doctor's office. You will need an appointment. But since the qualifying requirements vary widely, be sure to inquire about them in advance. Most importantly, do not confuse the hospital emergency room with the outpatient department. Although your breast lump seems a legitimate emergency to you, the emergency room staff just won't see it that way—anything that can wait a day or two is not an emergency to them. Since you'll be turned away from the emergency room, you might as well save yourself time and trouble by avoiding it altogether. Go directly to the outpatient department instead.

The American Cancer Society, some labor unions, and women's organizations frequently sponsor breast cancer screening clinics that travel from neighborhood to neighborhood and provide diagnostic testing, free of charge. These clinics are usually advertised in the sponsoring organization's newsletters and mailings, or in local newspaper articles and radio announcements. If you're looking for a way to get your annual breast examination, these temporary clinics are excellent. If you already have a lump, however, don't wait for the mobile screening clinic to come to your neighborhood. You must see a doctor immediately.

The American Cancer Society and the National Cancer Institute jointly operate twenty-seven breast cancer screening clinics around the United States. You'll find a directory of these clinics at the back of this book. But these screening clinics will test only women who do *not* have any symptoms of cancer—that is, you can get your annual checkup there, but you can't get a lump examined. However, if you call or write the center nearest you, they can refer you to a clinic that will take you if you already have a lump.

Making an appointment

Once you are armed with a list of telephone numbers, start calling. Tell the receptionist that you have never seen the doctor before (or been to the clinic before), but that you got his (its) name from the *Directory of Medical Specialists* (or, the county medical society, the American Cancer Society, or wherever). Then tell her that you have discovered a lump in your breast and fear it may be cancer. Insist on seeing the doctor right away.

Some women don't want to discuss their medical problems with anyone but the doctor, but in this case it is imperative that you tell the receptionist the facts. If you merely request an appointment for a physical, don't be surprised if she schedules you for two or three weeks later. Receptionists are not mind readers. Once she knows your problem, a good receptionist will juggle the doctor's appointments, if necessary, to fit you in within two or three days. If she insists that the doctor cannot see you within a few days, forget that doctor and call another one from your list. You need a doctor who is available.

If you are trying to get an appointment at a free clinic, or outpatient department, and the receptionist tries to put you off after she knows your problem, stand your ground. Ask to speak with the clinic director personally. You may have to dial the hospital switchboard and ask for the doctor by name (have him paged if necessary) to get to him, but keep at it until you do. No doctor will turn away a patient who has a lump in her breast; he'll figure out a way to get around the red tape and see you as soon as possible.

Keeping your appointment

As you have already discovered, doctor's appointments are not easy to come by. So be sure to keep your appointment. If you must cancel your appointment, be sure to call at *least* twenty-four hours in advance, or you may be charged for the missed appointment. If you cancel several appointments, the doctor may refuse to make any further ones for you; he will not continue to commit his time to a patient who never shows up. If you miss an outpatient clinic appointment, you may have to wait at least a week to see a doctor, since gynecology patients may be seen only one day a week.

What to expect

If this is your first visit to a new doctor, he will meet with you first in his personal office area. Here, while you sit across the desk from each other, the doctor will ask you a long list of questions about your health and your family's health. For example, he will ask you how old you are, when you had your last menstrual period, if you've ever had trouble with your breasts before, and so on.

Your answers to these questions constitute your medical history and help your doctor to determine just how high a risk you run of having breast cancer.

Next, the doctor's nurse will show you into the examining room. She will give you a gown to put on after you've removed your clothes. After you've had time to get ready, the doctor will come in to give you a complete physical examination.

First he looks in your eyes, ears, nose, and mouth. He gently feels around the top of your neck to see if your lymph nodes are swollen. Then he uses a stethoscope to listen to your chest as you breathe slowly and deeply. Of course, he will take your temperature, pulse, and blood pressure, too.

To examine your breasts, the doctor stands behind you and reaches around your chest to palpate (gently prod) your breasts, much the same way that we learned in Chapter Four. Still in this position, the doctor feels your upper chest and underarms for swollen lymph nodes. Then you lie down on your back, and the doctor examines your breasts again.

As you lie on your back, the doctor gently pushes and prods your abdomen as he looks for areas of tenderness. This is no time to be brave—if it hurts, say so. After the abdominal examination is completed, you place your feet in the stirrups of the examining table for the pelvic or internal examination.

To accomplish this, the doctor inserts a speculum into your vagina to hold the vaginal walls open; in this way he can see the entire inside of your vagina and the cervix, or entrance to the uterus or womb. If it has been a year or more since your last pelvic examination, the doctor will take a Pap smear to check for cervical cancer. This test is simple and painless; you probably won't even feel it. Next, the doctor inserts his gloved finger into your rectum to check for possible rectal cancers.

In addition, most doctors have a nurse remain in the examining room during the pelvic and rectal examinations. If your doctor does not call the nurse in, and you would prefer that she be there, you are perfectly right in insisting on her presence. Your doctor will be happy to comply.

Many women avoid a yearly checkup because they are embarrassed by or afraid of the pelvic examination. The only way to overcome these fears is to grit your teeth and go through with it. Millions of women have made it through the examination, and so will you. Your doctor anticipates your feelings; this is why he meets with you first in his office area where you can get to know him better and begin to build thrust in his professional attitude. The actual examination is accomplished as quickly and gently as possible.

Is your doctor right for you?

The prime factor in deciding if your doctor is the right doctor is the level of trust and confidence he inspires. If he doesn't seem to know what he is doing, or if he's slipshod about the physical examination, he's definitely not the right doctor. You need a doctor who is thorough and competent.

How can you know if he is competent? If you know and trust another doctor, you could ask him. But if you don't know anyone to ask, you'll have to rely on your own observations. Is the office clean? Are the receptionists and nurses helpful and sympathetic? Competent doctors usually try to surround themselves with competent office personnel.

Is the office well equipped? Does the doctor seem to be confident and efficient, to know what he is doing? Does he keep good records of your visits? A good record means an individual file folder with your name on it; inside are orderly sheets of paper with notes on your visits, lab and X-ray reports, and your medical history.

Still, a good doctor is not necessarily the *right* doctor. The doctor (family doctor or gynecologist) who is right for you should have these qualities in addition to his medical knowledge:

1. He should listen to you.

2. He should let you ask questions and he should answer them in language that you can understand.

3. He should care about you as a person and make sure you're informed about your condition.

4. When he feels a second opinion is needed, or whenever you express a desire for a second opinion, he is happy to call in another doctor (not his associate) for an objective judgment.

5. He should not proceed with a biopsy until all other nonsurgical means of diagnosis have been exhausted.

6. Should surgery be necessary, he does not attempt to do it himself; he calls in a qualified surgeon.

It is essential that your gynecologist puts your

best interests first when he makes a medical decision. This means that he must always consider your *personal feelings* about the matter in the same way that he considers his own knowledge and experience. Except in the area of medical expertise, you *are* the equal of your doctor. His attitude must reflect this equality. If he is patronizing or if he treats you only as a body and not as a human being, you don't need him as your doctor. Your body is yours, not his. The ultimate decision over what happens to your body is also yours.

Find out about his hospital

It's always a good idea to find out which hospital your doctor uses. After all, you may someday have to go there under emergency conditions. You need to know that your doctor practices at a good hospital.

A good hospital should be accredited by the JCAH (Joint Commission on Accreditation of Hospitals). This accreditation means that the hospital has voluntarily opened itself up to a thorough investigation by a team of doctors, nurses and hospital administrators. The accreditation certificate should be displayed prominently in the hospital lobby or near the administration office. If you're in doubt about a hospital's accreditation, you can write to:

Joint Commission on Accreditation of Hospitals
875 N. Michigan Avenue
Chicago, Illinois 60611

They'll be happy to answer your questions.

A hospital that serves as a teaching institution for medical students or interns and residents is usually topnotch. A hospital doesn't have to be near a medical school to be a teaching hospital. You can find out if there are any teaching hospitals near you by writing to:

The Council on Medical Education
American Medical Association
535 N. Dearborn Street
Chicago, Illinois 60610

If you want to know exactly how good a hospital is, you can go to the administrator's office and ask to see a copy of the hospital's vital statistics. The *total* death rate of all patients in the hospital should be no greater than 3%. The infant mortality rate should be no higher than 2%, and the maternal death rate no more than 0.25%.

Less than 1 in 5,000 patients undergoing surgery should die as a result of the anesthesia, and not more than 1% of all patients should die post-operatively (after surgery). Autopsies should have been performed on 20-30% of all the patients who died in the hospital. Consultations (second opinions from expert specialists) should be recorded for 15-20% of all hospitalized patients. No more than 3-4% of all patients should have complications arising from their treatments, and only 1-2% should have contracted infections while in the hospital. Pathology reports should confirm that no more than 10% of all tissues removed in surgery were disease-free.

By asking for these statistics, you run the risk of antagonizing the hospital administrator, but his momentary anger is a lot less important to you than how good his hospital is. Don't take no for an answer—you are entitled to see these statistics. A hospital that can match these figures is a good one.

Chapter Seven

IS IT CANCER?

Breast cancer cannot be diagnosed by physical examination alone. After your doctor examines your breasts, he compares his findings to the information contained in your medical history. Then, mainly on the basis of probability, he decides whether you need other, more reliable diagnostic examination.

For example, if you are fourteen years old and have breast lumps which appear only during your period, your doctor may want you to wait through another menstrual cycle to see if the lump will go away by itself. The laws of probability are overwhelmingly in your favor—you most likely have only a benign breast condition.

But if you are over thirty-five years of age, *or* if you have a family history of breast cancer, your doctor will probably want you to have further diagnostic examinations. He may order mammography, xerography, thermography, or a combination of these procedures.

Mammography is X ray of the breast. While not 100% accurate in distinguishing malignant tumors from benign ones, the X-ray procedure is very useful nevertheless. For women over the age of forty-five, for women with family histories of breast cancer, and for women whose breasts are difficult to examine because of their large size or lumpy texture, mammography is often used as a routine examination about every three years. For very young women, mammography is usually avoided, unless it is absolutely necessary, since no one knows what the results of repeated exposures to the X ray will be. The radiation dosage of one mammogram is extremely small; the potential danger lies in the cumulative effect of many exposures throughout a woman's lifetime—i.e., a build-up of radiation.

The mammography procedure itself is very simple. You sit before a special table upon which you rest each breast as it is X-rayed from above. Then you lie down on the table as each breast is X-rayed from a side view. Then each armpit is X-rayed. The X rays themselves are painless, but the compression technique (flattening of the breasts) necessary for good visualization, may be slightly uncomfortable to some women. Just be sure to hold your breath when the technician tells you to do so; if you breathe, the X-ray picture will be blurry.

Xerography (or xeroradiography) is essentially the same thing as mammography except that the picture is developed and printed differently. Most radiologists feel that the xerogram shows greater detail than the mammogram, but the equipment is expensive and not yet widely available. The procedure is more accurate than mammography for very young women, and about as accurate for everyone else. That is, there is an 80-90% accuracy rate, or a 10-20% error rate. The errors are usually false-positives: a lesion may be judged malignant on the xerogram and benign at biopsy. Occasionally, a false-negative result occurs, and a malignant (cancerous) tumor is falsely judged to be benign (harmless). This is why biopsies are done after the xerograms whenever there is any question as to the accuracy of the test or when the woman's family history is indicative of breast cancer.

Thermography, the third diagnostic examination for breast cancer, is not an X ray at all. Thermography is a measure of body heat; it is based on the idea that tumors produce more heat than do normal tissues. Unfortunately, this examination cannot differentiate between a malignant tumor and a benign tumor. It can only differentiate between a tumor and something else that does not produce excess heat, such as a cyst. For this reason, thermography is the least desirable of the three procedures described in this chapter.

Before a thermogram can be taken, you must sit with your breasts exposed and your arms held out away from your body for almost an hour; this waiting time allows your breasts to "cool down." Then, a heat sensitive device is passed over both breasts to determine the presence of any "hot spots." A positive thermogram should always be checked out further since there are a considerable number of false-positive results. You can have a hot spot and not have a tumor at all; breast infections, and even engorged milk ducts, produce heat that can show up as a suspicious hot spot on a thermogram. Any woman with a positive thermogram should also have a mammogram or xerogram as a double-check.

Of the three diagnostic examinations described in this chapter, xerography is preferred by most physicians. It is particularly valuable in detecting breast cancers that are too small to be felt as lumps. If xerography is not available in your community, then regular mammography will have to do. But be sure to find out how modern the X-ray equipment is. To do highly reliable mammography, a special molybdenum tube is necessary. Ask your radiologist if his equipment has such a tube. If it doesn't, find a doctor whose equipment is more up-to-date. There is no comparison between the old-fashioned mammography (without the molybdenum tube) and the modern technique.

No matter which examinations your doctor orders, you must call him to get the results. The radiologist cannot tell you the results himself because he does not have a copy of your medical history, or physical exam results, in front of him to compare with your X rays or thermogram. The radiologist describes what he finds to your own doctor, who then correlates the radiologist's findings with his own observations to arrive at a diagnosis. You should be able to get the results of your examinations from your gynecologist the next day, if not the same day.

While some breast lumps can immediately be diagnosed as cancerous or not on the basis of mammograms, xerograms, and thermograms, some lumps just cannot be diagnosed without a firsthand look. This actual look at the suspected cancer is called a biopsy. In the United States, the biopsy is most often performed in the operating room under general anesthesia. This procedure, and other biopsy techniques, will be discussed in the next chapter.

If your gynecologist feels you need a biopsy, he will refer you to yet another specialist. If you live in or near a very large city, this specialist may be a breast surgeon; but if you do not live near an urban center, the specialist may be a general surgeon, meaning that he does many kinds of operations on other parts of the body. Where one is available, an oncologist or cancer specialist may be called in to review the results of your X rays and to consult with the surgeon.

The biopsy operation has caused women immeasurable grief—not because of any technical difficulty with the biopsy itself, but because of the questionable practice of using a coercive consent form and subsequent drastic surgery without regard to the patient's wishes. In Chapter Eight, we'll examine this practice in detail and show you how you can avoid the problem.

surgeon must have your written, informed consent for the operation. "Informed consent" is supposed to insure that you understand exactly what will be done in the operating room. Instead, the present system of informed consent for breast biopsies accomplishes exactly the opposite; you're guaranteed *not* to know what has happened to you until you wake up afterward.

It is now standard procedure in the United States to offer the patient a combined consent form for both biopsy and mastectomy. (Mastectomy is the surgical removal of the breast, as described in Chapter Nine.) Your signature on this combined form gives your surgeon permission to *go ahead* with removal of the affected breast, if the lump is found to be malignant during the biopsy. The surgeon will not wake you up to tell you. In other words, you will have no idea when you go under the anesthesia whether you will wake up with one breast or two. The mental anguish of not knowing is totally unnecessary and unacceptable, especially when you consider that 65-80% of all the breast lumps biopsied are *not* cancerous. The majority of women undergoing surgical biopsy are suffering great mental anguish for nothing!

Even those women whose breast lumps are found to be malignant during the biopsy are not dealt with fairly if the surgeon goes ahead with the usual radical or modified radical mastectomy (see Chapter Nine). The quick diagnosis is made on what is called a frozen section. This means that a very thin slice of the tumor is quick-frozen and then placed under the pathologist's microscope. This doctor calls the specimen either malignant, benign, or indeterminate. If he says "malignant," the surgeon goes ahead with the mastectomy.

Later, when the patient is already back in her room, more samples of the tumor are stained with dyes for better viewing. The staining technique is very time-consuming, taking at least twenty-four hours to complete. Again the pathologist looks at the tumor under his microscope. This time he identifies the specific types of cancer cells present in the tumor and attempts to determine just how fast they reproduce themselves. He looks to see if the blood vessels or lymph channels have been invaded. Ideally, he should test the tumor for hormone dependence. This laboratory identification of the most minute details of the tumor, coupled with the results of your physical and X-ray examinations, is called "staging"; it helps your doctor decide whether you will need radiation therapy, chemotherapy, or hormone therapy after surgery, (see Chapter Eleven).

Tumor staging can also help determine just how much surgery is necessary, provided the surgeon is willing to do anything less than a radical or modified radical mastectomy. When the tumor is limited to the breast, less mutilative procedures may be employed (see Chapter Nine). It seems only logical to delay the choice of surgical method until all the details are clear and can be taken into consideration.

You may have some trouble finding a surgeon who is willing to go along with your plans for a separate biopsy procedure and treatment procedure. Until the last few years, the combination biopsy-mastectomy was not questioned; it has long been considered the only effective way to treat breast cancer.

Some doctors will argue that separate operations are risky because of the use of general anesthesia. While it is true that general anesthesia does carry a certain risk of death, that risk is only about one-in-five thousand. If you must have a surgical biopsy, then you must decide if you'd rather take that risk and know what's going to be done in the second operation, or if you'd rather not take the risk and not know before you go to sleep whether you'll lose your breast.

If neither choice sounds ideal (which it's not) you can press your doctor for a different kind of biopsy. It is standard practice in Great Britain to do an aspiration biopsy first. This involves insertion of a long hypodermic needle into the breast in an attempt to obtain some tumor cells for microscopic examination. The biggest advantage of this procedure is that it requires only local anesthesia and can be performed in the doctor's office. But, the procedure has one big disadvantage; it's too easy to get the needle in the wrong place and miss the tumor entirely. The doctor who performs an aspiration biopsy must be very skillful in the technique. Not many U.S. doctors are experienced enough in the procedure to rely on it for diagnosis.

Another simple biopsy technique involves the use of a wide-bore needle through which a tiny cutting instrument can be inserted to obtain a tissue sample of the tumor and its immediate surroundings. This procedure is more reliable than the aspiration biopsy and it can be performed under local anesthetic. This too is standard practice in Great Britain, but it hasn't caught on yet with American physicians. Ask your doctor about these procedures; he may be familiar with them or he may know someone else who is.

Another argument against the combined biopsy-mastectomy procedure becomes obvious when you consider that some women already have metastases by the time they discover their breast lumps or see a doctor. For these women, no breast operation, no matter how radical, is going to remove all their cancer. Why should they be subjected to a mutilating procedure for nothing? Simple studies called scans can detect metastases easily. If the stained pathology section reveals that the tumor is very advanced and fast-spreading, with evidence of blood vessel and lymph channel invasion, wouldn't it make sense to give the woman bone, brain, and liver scans and chest X rays to check for the presence of metastases? If there are metastases, simple removal of the tumor and chemotherapy and radiation treatments may be the best course of action (see Chapter Eleven).

Some surgeons may argue that a delay in surgical treatment after biopsy is dangerous because of the possibility that cancer cells will escape from the tumor through the surgical incision and start spreading throughout the body. There is absolutely no evidence that this happens. A two-day delay in surgical treatment after biopsy does not affect survival rates in the least. Besides, a breast cancer has

Chapter Nine

BREAST CANCER SURGERY: YOU *DO* HAVE A CHOICE

Throughout the world, various surgical techniques are used to treat breast cancer. In the United States, the radical, or Halsted, mastectomy has been used since 1894. Only recently have some surgeons taken up the modified radical mastectomy. In the rest of the world, simpler and less disfiguring operations are practiced. We'll examine each of these procedures in detail, but first let's review the normal anatomy of the chest.

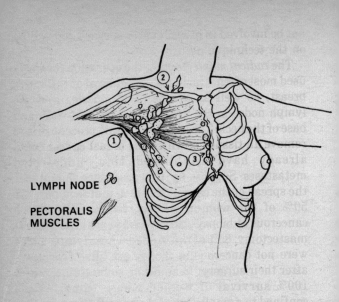

LYMPH NODE

PECTORALIS MUSCLES

As you can see in this diagram, the breasts are well supplied with lymph nodes. These nodes, as you recall, normally help to fight off disease; but they *can* become cancerous and then they contribute to the spread of the disease. There are three major chains of lymph nodes in the breast (numbered for you in the diagram): (1) those in the *axillae* or armpits, (2) those in the outer chest wall, between the pectoral muscles and continuing up to the base of the neck, and (3) those under the breastbone. The pectoral muscles (the major muscles of the chest) cover the rib cage and attach to the upper portion of the arm. All these structures may or may not be involved in breast cancer surgery, depending on the technique used.

The *radical mastectomy*—the operation formerly used most often—includes the removal of the entire breast, as well as the pectoral muscles and the lymph nodes in the armpits, outer chest wall, and base of the neck. The idea behind this procedure is to remove all tissues in which the breast cancer could already have established tiny, undetected metastases. Supposedly, this procedure should halt the spread of the cancer. But in actual fact, only 45-50% of the women whose lymph nodes were cancerous at biopsy still live five years after radical mastectomy; 85% of the women whose lymph nodes were not cancerous at biopsy are alive five years after their surgery. In addition, some studies claim 100% survival of women whose tumors were confined to a small area of the breast. Ten-year survival statistics are almost identical for all groups of women undergoing radical mastectomy. Unfortunately, the woman who has had this particular operation must wear high necklines to cover the hollows left in her upper chest. Sleeveless blouses cannot be worn because of the extensive scarring in the lower shoulder area and the underarm hollows.

The *extended radical mastectomy* is essentially the same procedure as the radical mastectomy, except that the lymph nodes under the breastbone are removed too. Generally, this operation is used only for women whose cancers are located on the inner side of the breast, toward the breastbone. Because of the extreme difficulty of removing the lymph nodes from beneath the breastbone, this operation should be done only by highly skilled surgeons in the best-equipped hospitals. The success rate of the extended radical mastectomy is about the same as that of the radical mastectomy. By the time the breast cancer has spread to these particular lymph nodes, it is usually too late to stop the spread of the disease, since there may already be metastases in other parts of the body. For this reason, the extended radical mastectomy is hardly ever justified.

The *modified radical mastectomy*—rapidly gaining in popularity among American surgeons—includes removal of the entire breast and the lymph nodes of the armpit, outer chest wall, and base of the neck. Surgeons who favor this operation believe that the pectoral muscles are not likely sites for metastases. The operation is somewhat more difficult to perform than the radical mastectomy, but the results are much less disfiguring. The range of arm motion possible after the modified radical mastectomy is somewhat greater too. Again, the five-year survival rates for the radical and modified radical operations are about the same. For very little risk, the patient gains the very big advantage of limited chest deformity; there is scarring in the chest and underarm, but there are no hollows in the chest.

The *simple mastectomy* is favored by physicians who believe that the more radical procedures slow down healing of the wound. This operation is simply the removal of the breast; the pectoral muscles and all lymph nodes are left in place. Theoretically, say the proponents of this operation, the lymph nodes should help the body fight off any cancer cells that remain after the operation. Should the lymph nodes later prove to be cancerous, they can be removed then. When simple mastectomy is followed immediately by radiation therapy, the combined procedure seems as effective as the radical mastectomy alone (in terms of five-year survival rates for women whose cancers are confined to the breast). Although the lymph nodes may not appear to be cancerous on physical examination, there is always the chance that they have already been invaded. Physical examination can be wrong. But reconstruction is almost always a possibility after simple mastectomy.

The *partial mastectomy* or *lumpectomy* involves removal of a very localized breast tumor and a small wedge of the tissue which surrounds it; most of the breast, the pectoral muscles, and the lymph nodes are left intact. Some surgeons who advocate this procedure cite cases in which one or two cancerous lymph nodes regressed (cleared up) after the breast tumor was removed. In any case, the lumpectomy is usually followed by radiation therapy in hopes of killing any other tiny cancers that might be present in the remaining breast tissue. There seems to be not much difference between the partial mastectomy or lumpectomy followed by irradiation, and the radical mastectomy alone, in terms of five-year survival rates when the cancer is strictly confined to the breast.

If all mastectomy procedures have the same five-year survival rates, then why don't surgeons abandon the radical and modified radical mastectomies, and perform only simple and partial mastectomies on women whose cancers are confined to the breast (and who have no evidence of lymph node involvement)? Most doctors believe that five-year survival rates don't mean much in themselves. A woman with breast cancer who goes untreated will usually live about four years after her cancer is diagnosed. Therefore, they argue, it is not too remarkable for a woman to survive five years after a simple or partial mastectomy. These doctors are waiting to see the ten-year survival figures for these two operations before they change their minds about which surgery is best.

But, unfortunately for American women, the simpler procedures just haven't been used long enough to obtain any long-term survival statistics. American doctors are sticking to their tried and true radical, and modified radical, procedures because at least they know what their patients' chances are with those procedures.

This "wait and see" attitude may soon be abandoned. A recent study by Dr. Barnard Fisher and his associates analyzes the long-term survival rates of women who have had radical mastectomies and emphasizes that the vast majority of women who had recurrences or metastases within ten years of their operations had them within five years. These researchers believe that five-year survival statistics offer sufficient evidence of long-term survival chances to be used in deciding which surgical procedure is most appropriate. However, the issue remains unsettled in the minds of most physicians.

As mentioned in the previous chapter, detailed examination of the biopsy specimen and thorough physical examination are necessary to determine whether the tumor is indeed confined to the breast. These findings should be confirmed with brain, bone, and liver scans and chest X rays. Only after all these examinations are completed should the surgeon make his recommendation of the type of surgery necessary.

The choice of surgical procedure is really up to you, the patient. Your surgeon cannot perform any operation on you for which you have not given your written, informed consent. Of course, you must depend on your doctor to take all factors into account and to make a thoroughly reasoned-through recommendation. Armed with the results of your pathology section examination, and the scans and X rays, you should be able to discuss alternative procedures with your physician.

For example, if your cancer is quite advanced and you already have metastases to other parts of your body, you may wish to forego surgery altogether—unless there is some indication that a combination of nonmutilative surgery and chemotherapy or hormone therapy will help you. Chapter Eleven describes the unpleasant side effects of these treatments which must also be taken into account when making your decision. If your cancer is of the very localized type, with no clinically evident invasion of the lymph nodes, you may want to have a lumpectomy; but remember that you take the chance that your lymph nodes might be cancerous. There is no 100% sure way of knowing unless the lymph nodes are removed and examined under the microscope. If your breast cancer has spread to the lymph nodes but you have no metastases, you may be very content to have the modified radical mastectomy.

In general, the procedure that is right for you depends upon the specific type of cancer you have; how fast it grows; whether or not you have cancerous lymph nodes or metastases; and how important your breasts are to you. If you would rather lose a breast than take a chance of having a recurrence, you may want to have the radical mastectomy. But you should keep in mind that even this type of extensive surgery is no guarantee that you won't have metastases. If your breasts are very important to you, you may prefer to start out with as simple a procedure as possible (provided your tumor is confined to the breast), and opt for careful and frequent monitoring for further evidence of cancer. You can have more radical surgery if and when you need it, but you take the chance that things could get out of hand before the recurrence or metastasis is discovered.

If you choose not to have the radical or modified radical mastectomy, prepare to meet some resistance. Some doctors feel that a woman has no business making decisions about her medical treatment; she must trust her doctor's decision totally. Other doctors just don't understand what all the fuss is about since they consider the breasts to be useless and easily disposable.

The sanest way to handle the mastectomy question is to choose a surgeon who you know will consider your feelings when recommending the type of surgery you should have. The truly humane surgeon considers you as a complete human being, and not as a breast cancer. He takes into account not only your cancer type but also your emotional make-up; he strives to suit the operative procedure to your individual needs.

If you are at all uneasy about your surgeon's recommendations, then by all means ask him or your gynecologist to call in another surgeon for an independent consultation. You will probably want to ask both doctors if they have ever performed either the simple or partial mastectomy and under what circumstances. If they have never performed either procedure and, even more importantly, do not foresee *any* circumstances under which they would perform them, then try to find yet another surgeon who has a more open mind. Whether you are paying the most expensive doctors in town, or you are depending upon free or low-cost resources for your medical care, you are entitled to a reasonable number of consultations before deciding whether to follow their advice.

When it comes time to sign the consent for your surgery, make sure you know what you're signing. Insist that the operation be described in writing, in terms you can understand. Remember, you can't take back your decision once the operation has been performed.

Chapter Ten

GOING THROUGH WITH IT

Don't be surprised if entering the hospital sends you into a state of panic. Most women do feel trapped and helpless once they're through the hospital doors. Some women even try to get their families to take them home in a last-ditch effort to avoid surgery. It is tempting. But you should bear in mind that 65-80% of all breast lumps biopsied are *not* cancer. The odds are in your favor.

The usual procedure is to check into the hospital the afternoon before your surgery is scheduled. Your surgeon will have arranged everything in advance, so the hospital admitting people will be expecting you.

Go first to the admissions office. There you'll have to complete some admissions forms that ask questions like: Where do you and your husband work? Do you have health insurance? If not, do you have credit references? If you do have health insurance (or Medicare or Medicaid) you'll need your policy or identification number, so be sure to bring it with you. In most hospitals you will be required to put up some kind of deposit if you don't have insurance. Your doctor can tell you in advance how much that deposit will be.

After all the forms are completed, you will be assigned to your room. You can choose a private room, a semi-private room (which you share with one person) or a ward (which you share with three or more patients). Most insurance policies will only pay for a ward or semi-private room; if you wish to have a private room you can expect to pay $20 a day or more out of your own pocket to make up the difference in price.

If you plan to share a room, be sure to tell the admissions clerk if you smoke or not. It is most unpleasant for a nonsmoker to share a hospital room with a chain smoker. It is equally unpleasant for a smoker to share a room with someone who's in an oxygen tent and therefore be forbidden to smoke.

A hospital volunteer will show you to your room. There you'll be met by a nurse who will show you where to put your things. Then you'll change into either your own nightgown or a hospital gown, whichever you prefer. The nurse will explain to you how to provide a urine sample for laboratory analysis.

After you've had a little time to settle in, you'll be visited by a laboratory technician. He or she will take a sample of your blood from a vein in your forearm. To the uninitiated, this looks like a gruesome procedure, but it's actually less painful than having your finger pricked. The tourniquet around your upper arm will make your entire arm feel slightly numb, but the numbness will go away within seconds after the procedure is completed.

You will also have a chest X ray and possibly an electrocardiogram (an ECG or EKG for short). These tests are given to make sure your lungs and heart are in good shape. If you have any fluid in your lungs or if your heart is weak, your doctor must know it now—before you're given inhalation anesthesia.

That evening, the anesthesiologist (the doctor who will administer the anesthetic for your operation) will drop by so that you can become acquainted. He'll be glad to explain to you exactly what type of anesthetic you will have and what it will be like. If you've ever had a bad experience with anesthesia before, be sure to tell him now so that he can avoid having the same problem this time. The doctor will order you not to eat or drink anything more until after you wake up from your operation. It is very important that you not have any food in your stomach when you are going to have a general anesthetic because of the danger that you will vomit while asleep and choke to death on your own vomit. If you're very dehydrated during the operation (and you will be if you don't drink any water the night and morning before), it will take less anesthetic to keep you asleep, and that is very much to your advantage.

The night before the biopsy is frightening to most women. It is always difficult to sleep in a strange place—especially when you're facing surgery in the morning. Patients harbor inside themselves a fear of not waking up from the anesthesia. Women who are about to have a breast lump biopsied are worried that the lump will be cancer.

Nightmares are common. One woman reported dreaming that when she went to the butcher shop she found hundreds of human breasts hanging from the meat hooks behind the counter. Don't be afraid that you are having a nervous breakdown if you have a dream like this. Your emotional health is better than that of the woman who denies the possibility of breast cancer and sleeps soundly through the night.

The next morning, you'll follow a prescribed pre-operative routine. If you are a smoker, your doctor may wish you to breathe through a special machine for a few minutes in order to clear out your lungs. This treatment is painless and is most easily carried out if you relax and breathe in rhythm with the machine.

A nurse will shave your chest and back and wash your breast with a germ-killing soap. Then you'll put on a sterile hospital gown and cap. (Your hair should be completely covered by the cap.)

Usually a sedative is administered to help you calm down before going to the operating room. These drugs affect people differently—that is, some people are virtually put to sleep by them while others are completely unaffected. If the injection does not make you woozy and you want to be "halfway out" before you get to the operating room, you can request another shot. In most cases the doctor has left orders that allow the nurse to give you a second shot, but it might be a good idea to prearrange this with your doctor, just in case. Finally, a member of the operating room staff will come for you with a guerney (table on wheels).

Once you're inside the operating room, you'll be transferred from the guerney to the operating table. Above you are big round lights; cabinets full of surgical supplies line the walls. The complicated-looking machines at your head will be used by the anesthesiologist to administer the anesthetic and to monitor your heartbeat and blood pressure during the operation.

Now the anesthesiologist begins his work. First he starts an I.V. (short for intravenous) by placing a short needle in a vein in your forearm or hand and taping the needle to your skin. Though the initial placement of the needle may cause a little pain, you won't be aware of it at all once it's taped into place. Flowing through this needle and into your body are the fluids that will help maintain your normal fluid balance during the operation. Soon the anesthesiologist adds the anesthetic to the fluid mixture, and you will go to sleep almost instantly. As you fall asleep you may be aware of the nurses painting your breast with antiseptic.

While you're asleep, your surgeon will remove the breast lump and a little of the surrounding tissue. He sends this tissue sample down to the pathology laboratory for microscopic examination. Then he sews up the wound and (provided you did not sign the combined biopsy-mastectomy consent form) you're sent to the recovery room.

The recovery room is an area where surgical patients stay until they wake up after their operations. There are enough registered nurses on duty here to keep a sharp eye on every patient. Once you wake up and your doctor has given his okay, you'll be wheeled back to your room and transferred into your bed.

The next day, after the tumor and tissue sample have been stained and examined under the pathologist's microscope, you'll find out your diagnosis. Don't bother using your bedside telephone to call the pathology lab for the results because they won't tell you. Neither will the nurses assigned to your case. Only your own doctor can give you the results, no matter which way they go.

If your lump was benign, then rejoice! You're home free—or at least you will be as soon as your doctor signs your release papers. Small-breasted women may be allowed to go home that afternoon. But if you have large breasts your doctor may want you to stay in the hospital one more day for observation since there is some chance that you will develop a hematoma, a painful puddle of blood beneath your incision. A brief period of rest after biopsy reduces the chances of developing a hematoma.

But if your lump was malignant, you and your doctor will have to discuss what kind of surgery is best for you and come to a decision. You'll sign a second consent form, and your mastectomy will be scheduled for the earliest possible time. Again, you'll not be allowed to eat or drink the night before the operation.

The morning routine will be exactly the same as it was for the biopsy, except that the type of anesthetic will be a little different. After you've fallen asleep, the anesthesiologist will insert a tube into your mouth and down into your trachea (the top of your breathing system). Through this tube—which you won't feel at all—you'll be breathing a gaseous anesthetic that will put you into a much deeper sleep. Then the surgeon goes ahead with the agreed-upon operation (see Chapter Nine). Since the radical mastectomy is the most painful, we'll use that for our example when discussing postoperative care and recovery. If you have a modified, simple, or partial mastectomy, your recovery will be somewhat easier.

The very first thing you will feel when you regain consciousness after surgery is profound anger. You will hate your doctor for taking your breast. You will hate yourself for getting breast cancer. You will even hate your husband for trying to be nice about it. All these feelings result from your wounded vanity and are completely normal. In fact, these hateful feelings are so common that they deserve a chapter to themselves. Therefore, a more detailed discussion of the psychological aspects of mastectomy is delayed until Chapter Twelve. Here let's discuss only the physical aftereffects of the operation.

The second thing you feel when you wake up after

a mastectomy is the numbness. The entire operated side of your chest will feel numb and tingly, the way your foot feels when it falls asleep. Next you're aware of the drainage tubes that stick out of the bandages and connect with a vacuum pump. These tubes allow excess blood and lymph to drain away from the wound site. You may find the tubes painful—some women do and some don't. Most report a sort of burning sensation until the tubes are removed on the third or fourth day. Once the tubes are removed, you'll feel only a painful tightness in your chest as if constant pressure were being exerted on your rib cage.

Your doctor will leave orders for pain and sleep medications with the nurses in case you should need them. If you're in pain, call the nurse and ask for medication. On the other hand, if she offers you a sleeping pill and you really don't want to sleep, you don't have to take it. You can set the pace when it comes to taking these medications.

Those of you who haven't had major surgery in the past ten years will be surprised to find that the nurses will insist that you get up and walk to the bathroom that afternoon. Yes—you'll be walking the very day of your surgery. Early walking is essential to a speedy recovery since moderate activity promotes healing. You will also be required to wiggle your fingers and do other small hand and arm movements to promote drainage of excess fluids from the incision site.

As soon as your doctor okays it, you'll be visited by a volunteer from the American Cancer Society's Reach to Recovery Program. This volunteer has recovered from a mastectomy herself, so she can answer almost any nonmedical question you have about adapting to your surgery. If you have not been visited by a Reach to Recovery volunteer within three or four days after your operation, be sure to mention it to your doctor.

The volunteer will give you a Reach to Recovery kit that includes a small rubber ball and a plastic-coated rope that you'll need for your exercises, and a very light temporary prosthesis (breast form) that you can pin inside your nightgown over the bandages. Also included is a list of stores where you can buy a permanent prosthesis when you're ready for it. Be sure to get her telephone number so you can call her later; you'll think of many more questions for her to answer within the next few months. She will call on you periodically to see how you're doing too.

One of the first exercises you'll learn utilizes the small rubber ball that was included in your Reach to Recovery kit. Hold the ball in the palm of your hand and squeeze it repeatedly, as shown in Figure 1.

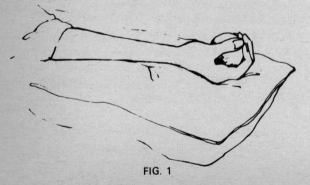

FIG. 1

At about the same time in your recovery, you can start brushing your hair and washing your face—with your weak arm, of course. Just be sure to hold your head erect. If you bend your neck to the side, you'll automatically rotate your wrist inward, and this movement can cause severe stress and pain in your armpit. The right and wrong ways to brush your hair are shown in Figure 2.

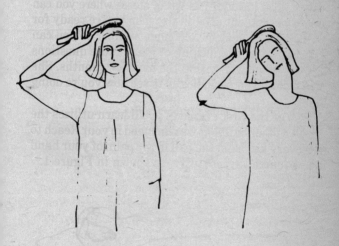

CORRECT

INCORRECT

FIG. 2

At times you will feel like using your hairbrush to hit the nurse or physical therapist over the head. The exercises can be painful and frustrating, but they are necessary. Exercising helps your recovery in two ways. First, it trains the muscles of your arm to take over the functions that your pectoral muscles used to do. And second, exercise promotes drainage of body fluids out of the arm and back toward the heart; this helps to prevent painful swelling of the arm. You must keep trying, no matter how frustrated you become.

If your arm does swell, it will help to elevate the arm by resting it on pillows. Sometimes an elastic bandage or sleeve is necessary when the swelling is very severe. But the best thing you can do is to prevent the swelling by keeping up with your exercises.

In the next few days you'll begin to do more strenuous exercises. As soon as your wound is healing nicely (and this event is marked by the beginning of a very annoying itch) you'll relearn how to rotate your arm by turning your palm upward and then downward again. This sounds like awfully slow going, and it is. But within a month or two, you'll have completely normal function of your arm—provided you *don't overdo it* now and cause your incision to reopen. Take it slow and easy, doing the exercises only as often as your doctor recommends.

By the time you're just about ready to leave the hospital (usually seven to ten days after mastectomy), you can progress to five more exercises. The simplest is the sideward raise exercise shown in Figure 3. To do this stand straight with arms hanging down at your sides. Now raise both arms straight outward until they're at shoulder level. Be careful not to bend your elbows.

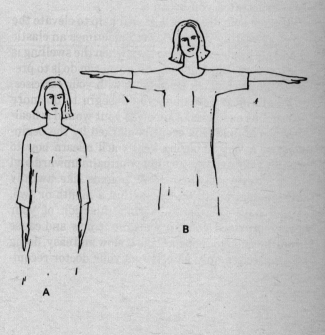

FIG. 3

Figure 4 demonstrates the stick exercise, another way to retrain your muscles. You'll need a short stick or the cardboard core from a roll of paper towels. Hold the stick with both hands in front of you at about thigh level. Then slowly swing your arms upward, keeping your elbows straight, until the stick is over your head.

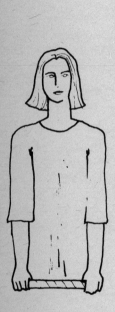

A

B

FIG. 4

You'll also need to learn the hand wall-climbing exercise or the "spider climb." To do this, stand facing the wall with both palms pressed flat against the wall at about shoulder level. Use your fingers to "walk" both hands up the wall until your arms are fully extended, as shown in Figure 5.

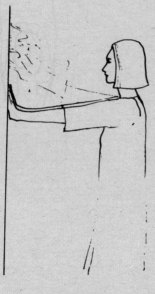

FIG. 5

The bra-fastening exercise is helpful too. Stand with your hands on your hips. Next, reach backward until your thumbs just brush the bottom of your shoulder blades—as if you were fastening your bra. See Figure 6.

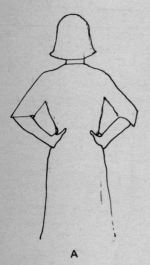

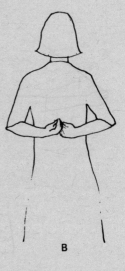

A   B

FIG. 6

You'll probably learn the pulley exercise shown in Figure 7, the last thing before leaving the hospital. You will need the plastic-covered rope that was included in your Reach to Recovery kit. Use your good arm to throw the rope over the shower curtain rod. Then hold one end of the rope in each hand. In this position you can slide the rope back and forth in a seesaw motion over the rod.

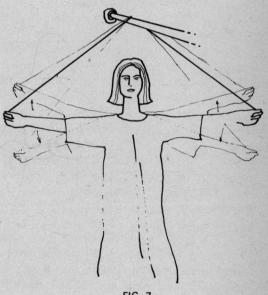

FIG. 7

Your doctor will tell you exactly which exercises to do and when you should do them. Do *not* start any of the exercises without your doctor's permission— but once you do start them, be sure to keep up with your exercises even after you go home.

Discharge from the hospital is an emotional experience. You're happy to be getting out of the hospital and returning to your family, but at the same time you wonder how you will ever manage at home. It will be helpful if your husband, a friend, or a relative can come to the hospital a little early to take care of the business details of checking out of the hospital. At this time, your insurance papers should be in order. If you don't have insurance you'll be required to make further payment on your bill and to arrange just how you're going to handle the rest of it. While all this is going on, you should try to rest so you won't be quite so tired out by the trip home.

You will need someone to drive you home, since you shouldn't drive for at least two weeks after your operation. But within three to four weeks you should be able to drive (provided your car has power steering) and participate in simple household activities. Within one or two months, your arm should be back to normal, with the possible exception of some remaining numbness under your arm. You can go back to all your normal activities, including sports, within three months after a radical mastectomy.

There are a few things which you must *not* do,

however. Never allow your arm on the operated side to be used for injections or blood tests, or for blood pressure readings. Don't wear tight rings or bracelets or even elasticized sleeves on that arm. You should avoid excessive weight gain and should not take hormones (including birth control pills) without your doctor's prescription.

If you should injure your arm in any way, attend to it immediately. Even if it's only a small cut or even a sunburn, it can become serious if not treated right away. Anytime your arm becomes infected, excess fluids accumulate under the infection site and cause your arm to swell. Once the swelling is there, it's very difficult to get rid of, so you are much smarter to avoid injury in the first place.

Some of your stitches may be removed before you leave the hospital, but most of them will have to wait at least another week to come out. Stitch removal doesn't hurt a bit and it signals a very important step in your recovery. Now that your incision has healed, you can probably start wearing a more natural prosthesis.

Your doctor will give you a prescription for your permanent prosthesis. Many kinds are available. Some are filled with a thin fluid and some are filled with a thick gel of silicone. Others are inflatable and some are even made of foam rubber. You will have to actually try them on in order to decide which style suits you best. If you like, your Reach to Recovery volunteer can help you pick out a prosthesis that will suit you.

Chapter Sixteen contains a directory of prosthesis manufacturers. You can write to these companies to find out the name of the store nearest your home that carries breast forms. Or you can look in the yellow pages of your telephone book under the heading "Artificial Breasts." Most stores that carry the prostheses have women who are especially trained to fit the breast forms to your unique needs; some of them will even come to your home for the fitting.

The most important thing in choosing a prosthesis is to take your time. At first you will probably be most comfortable wearing an unweighted breast form. Later, when your wound is entirely healed and your muscles are a little stronger, you'll probably want a weighted prosthesis that will help you maintain good posture.

If you have health insurance, Medicare, or Medicaid, be sure to have your receipt for your first breast form marked "surgical" so that it will be, at least in part, covered as a prescription item.

Some small-breasted women who already wear heavily padded bras or "falsies" may wish to continue this practice rather than buy an expensive prosthesis. This is fine, but a word to the wise—department store clerks are not used to seeing the scars of mastectomy and may recoil in horror. If this should happen to you, try to chalk it up to the clerk's ignorance. Don't let the insensitive reaction of an unimportant stranger affect your image of yourself. The first time it happens, you will probably not be able to take it so lightly, but you must learn to think in those terms if you are going to adjust to your new appearance.

Chapter Eleven

ADDITIONAL TREATMENTS

While mastectomy is an effective weapon against breast tumors and cancerous lymph nodes, surgery on the breast does not destroy those cancer cells that have already escaped into the bloodstream and lymph channels. Seventy-six percent of all women whose lymph nodes were positive at biopsy, and who were treated with mastectomy alone, have treatment failures (recurrences and/or metastases) within ten years of their surgery; 25% of the women whose lymph nodes were not cancerous, and who were treated with mastectomy alone, have treatment failures within ten years. This is why other related treatments are usually given as preventive measures. Chemotherapy, hormone therapy, and radiation therapy are very effective in preventing further cancers.

Chemotherapy (that is, drug treatments with such chemicals as 5-fluorouracil, cytoxin, predni-sone, or diethylstilbestrol) is often used to kill cancer cells that are freely circulating with the blood and lymph. These treatments may be in the form of injections or pills, both being equally effective. Unfortunately, there are a few very un-pleasant side effects of these drugs; you may become nauseated and have recurring vomiting and diarrhea; you may lose some or all of your hair and develop sores in your mouth. These side effects are *not* due to an overdose of the drugs, so *do not* reduce the amount you are taking without consulting your doctor first. You must remember that the whole idea of chemotherapy is to kill the cancer cells before they can kill you. This requires very powerful drugs. The nausea, vomiting, and mouth sores are temporary. The hair loss can be permanent, but can easily be covered with a natural-looking wig. Most women consider these unpleasant side effects to be minor compared to the alternative (breast cancers usually metastasize to the bones and there cause excruciating pain). However, this is something each woman must decide for herself.

Hormone therapy is often used to control the growth of cancers that have already metastasized. If your tumor was shown to be hormone dependent at biopsy, and you show signs of recurrence or metastases, your doctor may suggest that you have your ovaries removed (oophorectomy or ovariectomy). His suggestion is based on the knowledge that many breast cancers are dependent upon the presence of the female hormone estrogen for growth. Removal of the ovaries brings estrogen production to a halt and in 25-40% of all cases brings about a remission—that is, the growth rate of cancer cells is greatly slowed down or even stopped completely—for up to one year. If you show a positive response to the oophorectomy but that response wears off, your doctor may suggest that you have your adrenal glands removed (adrenalectomy), or possibly even have your pituitary gland removed (hypophysectomy). These operations bring about a remission of one to two years in 30-40% of the cases.

Oophorectomy, adrenalectomy, and hypophysectomy act to change hormone balance by removing the sources of estrogen production. But there is another way to alter hormone balance: doctors can administer other hormones to counteract the effects of the undesirable hormones. For example, if a woman's tumor is estrogen dependent (it depends upon the presence of the female hormone, estrogen, to grow), then androgens, or male hormones, can be administered to counteract the estrogens. This treatment is about 20% effective in bringing about remission that may last up to one year. Conversely, if the woman's tumor is androgen dependent, it can be treated with estrogens. Estrogen therapy is 36-40% effective in bringing about a remission of up to two years' duration.

But even these very effective treatments are not without side effects. Androgen therapy can cause masculinization complete with deepening of the voice, acne, persistent facial flush, and an increased sex drive. Estrogen therapy can cause vaginal bleeding, darkening of the areola (the skin around the nipple), breast pain, gastric disturbances, and difficulty in controlling urination. Both hormone therapies can cause hypercalcemia—or calcium deposits in the kidneys, lungs, and heart—and edema, or swelling resulting from salt retention.

The treatment most commonly used in conjunction with mastectomy is radiation therapy. X rays are effective killers of immature cancer cells, and are often used after mastectomy to kill any cancer cells that were not removed during the operation. Theoretically, this makes sense; but there is currently quite a controversy over the use of radiation therapy as a routine procedure after radical mastectomy. Some doctors believe that irradiation actually encourages the growth of metastases because it decreases the efficiency of the immune response.

There is no getting around the fact that radiation therapy can be most unpleasant. There is no pain during the actual treatments, but the side effects that come later can seem unbearable. Early in the course of treatment, the wound site may become red and swollen. The arm on the operated side may become so swollen with retained fluids that movement of the arm is difficult. (Should this occur, your doctor will prescribe a series of exercises that will help to minimize the condition.) Soon the skin around the wound becomes darker in color as the amount of pigment in the skin increases in response to irradiation—a sort of exaggerated suntan effect. The surface layers of the skin become dry and start peeling; the underlayers may become stringy and begin to form raised, bumpy, reddish blotches. The surgical wound may ooze a yellowish liquid. During this period, any sudden movement can cause the wound to reopen so that further stitching is required. Since the radiation field(the area exposed during radiation therapy) is much larger than just the incision, the mid-chest is affected too: structural changes in the esophagus may make swallowing difficult and a dry, hacking cough may develop.

Since there is no appreciable difference in the survival rates of women who undergo irradiation immediately after radical mastectomy and those who start radiation treatments only after an actual recurrence, it seems only logical to wait. Why suffer through the undesirable side effects of radiation therapy when you may never have a recurrence at all? But this reasoning applies only to women who have the radical mastectomy.

If you have the modified, simple, or partial mastectomy, you must have radiation therapy right away since in these less radical surgeries, tissues are left behind that have a very high chance of harboring tiny, as yet undetected, cancers. Radiation and chemotherapy can kill these immature cancers without further surgery. The wound will heal much faster with these operations, so radiation begun just a few days after surgery is actually started after the wound has already begun to heal. The danger, and discomfort, of the wound reopening is minimized.

Radiation has an overwhelmingly good effect when breast cancer is far advanced and has already spread to the bones. In this case, the prime goal of irradiation is relief of pain, and it is very effective in this regard. At the same time, the bones are strengthened. This is very important since a cancerous bone breaks very easily. A collapsed vertebra (one of the small bones of the spine) can cause paralysis of both legs, so irradiation is obviously very valuable as a preventive measure in these cases.

These additional therapies—chemotherapy, hormone therapy, and radiation therapy—have their good points and their bad points, as you have seen. You doctor may recommend any or all of these treatments to you; but again, the ultimate decision is yours. Do the possible bad effects outweigh the possible good effects? Would you rather undergo irradiation now (after radical mastectomy) or wait out an actual recurrence? How much uncertainty can you tolerate? These are questions that you and your doctor should discuss before you start any of the treatments outlined in this chapter. Remember that you're the one who suffers through the bad effects, as well as the benefits from the good effects. That makes it *your* decision.

Chapter Twelve

WHY AM I SO DEPRESSED?

The paradox of a patient cured of breast cancer but made emotionally ill by the cure has only recently been recognized as a legitimate medical problem. Although medical journals have been filled with reports of post-mastectomy depression for many years, too many doctors have failed to realize just how seriously the patient suffered. Patients were not warned that emotional problems might follow mastectomy. When the unsuspecting patient told her doctor of her terrible depression, he would come up with some statement like: "I saved your life. What else do you want?"

Fortunately, the medical profession is finally

beginning to realize that postoperative depression is the most common complication of mastectomy. Most women react to the loss of a breast with the same sadness they would feel when faced with the loss of a loved one or even a beloved object—like wedding photographs, for example. This very natural feeling of extreme sadness and over-whelming awareness of the missing person or item is called "object loss depression." Amputees feel the same kind of depression after losing a limb. Almost every woman who undergoes the operation suffers some resulting depression, ranging from simple listlessness to suicide. How can you tell if you're on the road to severe depression? Let's examine the symptoms of depression: lack of energy, disinterest, worry, insomnia, anxiety, nervousness, and pain.

Lack of energy in the first month or so after surgery is quite natural—no woman is going to feel like running around the block the day she gets home from the hospital. But within a few months she should feel like resuming most of her old activities. If, after some months, the woman cannot drag herself out of bed in the morning, or if she spends her entire day just sitting and doing nothing, her chronic state of fatigue is probably a sign of depression. Lack of appetite, weight loss, and recurrent constipation accompanying the fatigue also indicate depression.

People who are depressed often find that they no longer enjoy the activities that previously gave them great pleasure. When watching her children at play, a depressed mother may be overly critical and find it impossible to tolerate their happy noises.

Some women refuse to see their old friends because it's just too much trouble to get ready for visitors or to go visiting themselves. Working women often find it difficult to concentrate on the job; their memory lapses are really due to depression.

Apprehension and fear over the outcome of day-to-day activities is also a sign of depression. The woman recuperating at home may worry each day that her husband will be in an automobile accident on his way home from work, for example. Crying over the death of someone who died years before is common, too.

Almost all depressed people have sleep problems, either not sleeping enough or sleeping too much. Some patients have trouble falling asleep; others can fall asleep easily when they first go to bed, but they wake up in the middle of the night and are unable to go back to sleep. Usually this sort of insomnia can be linked to bad dreams and nightmares. Some depressed patients sleep all the time, but they never feel rested. Psychiatrists theorize that these people sleep to avoid having to face their problems.

Anxiety, another symptom of depression, differs from fear in its "specificity." A fear can generally be linked to a specific cause or object of that fear—fear of high places, fear of getting fat, etc. Anxiety, on the other hand, is not at all specific. The anxious person is nervous, uneasily expecting some impending doom. "Something terrible is about to happen," she thinks, but she has no idea what that terrible something could be. She weeps easily, having no idea why she cries.

All mastectomy patients experience pain. But the depressed woman has constant pain that lasts months. Sometimes the pain moves around inside her body—first it's in her back, then her legs, then her stomach. Her pain goes far beyond the normal post-surgical pain.

What are the real causes of post-mastectomy depression? The causes are complex and may vary at different stages of recovery. Upon awakening after the operation, most women report an over-whelming feeling of humiliation. They feel like mutilated freaks, desexed and repulsive. Too often, women feel that the loss of a breast is a punishment for some real or imagined misdeed. "I loved my body too much," they lament. Or "I know God is punishing me for my past adultery." Of course this kind of thinking is nonsense, but patients under the influence of anesthetics and sedatives are not known for their rationality.

Later, when the mind-numbing, pain-killing drugs have worn off, the more precise fears and doubts are expressed. Foremost among these fears is the realization of one's own vulnerability. Some-how we all convince ourselves that bad things can-not happen to us—they always happen to someone else, right? The woman who has just lost a breast to cancer can hardly believe that she is invulnerable; she must give up this self-deception.

"When I realized that cancer *was* happening to me I suddenly realized that bad things could happen to my family too," Helen J. remembers. She began to worry about them: "I was sure that my husband would be killed on the freeway and that my son

would fall off the jungle-gym and get a concussion."
Helen became the proverbial mother hen, hovering
over her family in an attempt to protect them from
harm. Other women faced with the same situation
simply withdraw from their family and friends,
fearing to become more emotionally involved.
Somehow, they think, this withdrawal makes them
less open to future pain in case a loved one should
become ill, hurt, or die.

All women who get breast cancer ask, "Why me?"
Most even discover within themselves jealous and
hateful feelings toward women they formerly merely disliked. "There's this woman who works in my
office who really *deserves* to get cancer." Janice's
laugh is sarcastic and bitter. "I mean she smokes
like a chimney and has for twenty years. But does
she get cancer? She doesn't even have smoker's
cough. *I'm* the one who ends up with cancer. It just
isn't fair!"

Janice is right—it isn't fair. But Janice would be
wise to remember that life doesn't offer any
guarantees. Innocent people are killed by drunk
drivers every day. The realization that life is unfair
is *not* a sign of depression; it's an accurate
observation of reality. But the woman who finds
herself *dominated* by her hateful feelings toward
women who are healthy, is severely depressed.

Since most people associate the word "cancer"
with a slow and painful death, it is only natural that
mastectomy patients are very much afraid of dying.
The threat of death is so everpresent that some patients actually find themselves preparing to die.
They may take positive action, like making out a

will; or negative action, like refusing to buy any new clothes. They also develop an entirely new speech pattern that is death-oriented. "After I'm gone," "When I die," and "I can't make plans that far in advance," become standard phrases.

While her chest is still covered with bandages, it's tempting for the mastectomy patient to pretend that the operation never happened. Some women actually manage to blot it out of their memories despite the pain of the incision. But when the bandages come off, the mastectomized woman can no longer deny reality—she is different, she has only one breast.

Despite many doctors' contention that the breasts are not needed after the child-bearing days are over, to most women, the loss of a breast represents a drastic change in their feminine orientation. In this country, breasts have both an *actual* use and a *symbolic* use: the actual use is the nursing of babies, and the symbolic use is sexual allurement. Let's face it—we live in a breast-oriented society. Movies and television flaunt beautiful heroines in plunging necklines. Topless dancers and waitresses are now standard for bars and lounges. Teenagers go braless and wear see-through blouses. In the face of such fierce competition for her husband's attention, the woman who has had a mastectomy is understandably insecure about her sexuality. If her husband finds it difficult to accept his wife's altered appearance and fails to resume sexual relations, adjustment is extremely difficult.

The woman who judges others largely on the basis of physical appearance has an especially difficult problem; she will be extremely harsh in her judgment of herself. She considers an incomplete body the same as an incomplete person. When a woman's feelings of self-worth, of completeness as a woman and as a human being, are centered around her body, mastectomy is bound to cause severe depression.

All of us wage inside us a continual war of dependence versus independence—that is, we like to think we can take care of ourselves, but we also enjoy having someone around to take care of us. When we're sick, this dependence/independence conflict really comes to the fore. It's comforting to have nurses, friends, and family waiting on us hand and foot, but at the same time it makes us feel a little incompetent. Some things we'd really rather do for ourselves. That's why we sometimes yell at someone who is only trying to help.

Of course, different people react to sickness in different ways. Some women resume their household duties as soon as possible after surgery—sometimes too soon. In their haste to reestablish their independent lifestyle, they inadvertently cause their wounds to reopen, and thus end up back in the totally dependent stage once again. Other women become stuck in the initial dependent stage, doing nothing for themselves and preferring to have others take care of them. This is all right for the first month after surgery, but it becomes silly after two or more months.

We have further dependence/independence conflicts in regard to our families. "I worried, before the surgery, how my husband and children would survive while I'm in the hospital," Sherry N. says. "But when I saw that they were getting along just fine without me, I felt like they didn't need me at all. I thought I'd been deceiving myself all these years." In extreme cases, the woman may believe that her family does better without her, and so she begins to make plans to do away with herself.

The temptation to step out of the picture is strongest for women whose families have severe financial problems, especially when the woman herself has been the main source of family income. If her cancer is advanced and she is unable to work, she soon sees her financial role changing from provider to consumer, and soon there is no money left either to pay mounting medical bills or buy food for the family. Because her thinking is distorted by her depression, she may decide that her family is better off without her.

What can you do if you find that you are sinking into this kind of depression? You *cannot* handle it by yourself; you *must* seek help. The logical people to ask for help are the surgeon who performed your mastectomy, your gynecologist, or your minister. They can refer you to the proper source of help through either group or individual psychotherapy. Don't worry if you cannot afford to pay. There are many free mental health clinics that are operated by community agencies. Your doctor can tell you where to find help.

One source your doctor might recommend is the American Cancer Society's Reach to Recovery Program. As mentioned in Chapter Nine, these women have recovered from mastectomies themselves.

Any time you're feeling down, you can call a Reach to Recovery volunteer who will help you get over the rough spots. She'll be glad to share your feelings and to help you in any way she can.

The most important part of dealing with any help source is remembering your goal, to learn to live with reality. Some insensitive people will offer you such ridiculous advice as "Go to the beauty shop and get a new hairdo" or "Why don't you go out and buy yourself a new dress?" Obviously, a new hairdo and a new dress won't make your breast grow back. Nothing will do that. Your best plan of action is to work actively toward a new self-realization, a new self-concept.

Instead of remaining passive and letting things happen to you, try being active—*start happening to things*. Sound impossible? It's not; in fact, it's really quite easy. Try thinking of your body in different terms: instead of considering your body as identical to your real self, consider it as only the vehicle that your real self uses for transportation. Your real self is made up of all those intangible qualities of your character that make you a unique human being— your generosity, your concern for others, your understanding, your ability to encourage your children to independence.

If you are a religious person, you might think of your real self as your spiritual self. Women who are not religious must at least accept the fact that there is a part of everyone that is separate from the physical body. Doctors can explain just which parts of the brain control our breathing and speaking, but they have yet to discover what controls our personalities or what makes each person a completely unique individual. Even identical twins, who are exactly alike in physical appearance and who developed from exactly the same genetic material, often have completely different personalities and attitudes.

Your real self is all those things that make you a unique person and therefore invaluable to family and friends. They don't love you for your body. They love you because you make them feel loved.

Because they do love you, you can talk about your problems with them. If they're doing something that really aggravates you, or if they fail to do something that you need them to do, tell them. You might say, "I really appreciate your wanting to help me around the house. But exercise is good for me right now. I need to learn how to use my arm again. I know it will take me longer to do it myself, but I'd really like to do it anyway. If you would like to help me, though, you could return these books to the library for me." In this way you can let your family and friends know that you appreciate their help, but you can redirect their energies toward activities that are acceptable to you both.

Remember that your friends want to help you, but often they just don't know how to go about it. Help them to help you by explaining your situation to them. For example, if you find yourself shouting at a friend for no good reason, you can say, "I'm sorry I shouted at you. I've been feeling depressed and angry at the world lately. My outburst had nothing to do with you. I really love you and I

You, the friend or relative, must try to understand how she feels in order to be able to help her.

Have you ever wondered how a baby feels as he lies there all alone in his crib? Do you think he wonders what all those strange and powerful people will do to him next? If you can imagine the baby's feelings, you may be close to understanding what the mastectomized woman feels like. Strangers have been taking care of her in the hospital; they took her breast and left her scarred for life. They forced her to do painful exercises when she felt more like just lying there and crying. Now that she's home, she wonders if her family and friends will further punish her; will they abandon her because she did the wrong thing (got cancer) and is now a "one-breasted freak" because of it?

The tiny, frightened baby and the woman who has just had a mastectomy have a common need—the need for stability and security. How can you help to satisfy that need? You can say over and over, in as many ways as you can think of, that you love her and will always love her, no matter what. The mastectomized woman needs to let go, to cry, to grieve over her loss without fear of rejection.

Your first step in demonstrating unconditional love is to recognize the realities of her mastectomy. Friends and relatives who pretend that nothing has happened are no help at all. Neither are people who lavish cooing attention and constantly help the woman, keeping her a cripple; they are actually hurting her by encouraging her to remain dependent and childlike. Time and time again, women report that they were helped most by their friends and relatives who faced the situation head on.

"Pat, my best friend, really got me through the whole thing," Anna K. remembers. "She cried with me when I saw my scars for the first time. Later, she helped me go through all my clothes to pick out the ones I could still wear. When I really got to feeling sorry for myself, Pat would tell me how glad she was to have me for a friend. Can you imagine that? Here she was knocking herself out for me, and she's telling me what a great friend I am! I don't know what I would have done without her."

Anna's friend Pat just reacted naturally, the way that children do. Children worry that their mother is suffering, that the incision is painful; but mostly, children are glad to have their mother back home. More importantly, the kids tell her so. Their need for mothering overcomes any anxieties they have about her surgery. Don't husbands have just as strong a need to have their wives back home? Don't friends feel joyous when their friend is back in their midst? Simple expression of these natural feelings is all that's needed. A loving "I need you so much" or a cheery "I'm so glad you're back home" reassures the mastectomy patient that her life *will* get back to normal.

Pat also helped Anna by exhibiting empathy instead of sympathy. Sympathy means "I feel sorry for you" and carries with it a silent but understood "and I'm so glad it was you who got the cancer and not me." Empathy, on the other hand, means "I feel your pain. When you're sad, I'm sad. When you're happy, you make me happy too." Pat accepted Anna's disfigurement as a hurting experience, but she made it clear that the surgery had not altered their friendship.

"My husband was really great," Marjorie R. smiles as she tells her story. "From the first week or so after I came home from the hospital, Bob was careful to include me in everything—and I do mean everything. Saturday mornings have always been our big clean-up days. The first Saturday I was home, Bob assigned me to dust the piano keys. It was really difficult because my arm hurt all the time. When I gave up and tried to beg off, Bob gave me a very stern lecture. 'No way,' he said. 'Everybody has to do his part around here and today the piano keys are your part.' I was never so happy to dust the piano keys in all my life!"

Bob's gentle humor helped Marjorie to accept that her contribution to the household workload was temporarily limited. But at the same time he left it open for Marjorie to take on other tasks as she felt like it. She could accept his help without feeling guilty because he maintained a good-natured attitude about his increased workload.

A husband or lover truly has the greatest opportunity to help, especially when the bandages are removed for the first time. At that moment, the woman does not look at her wound; she looks at her husband's face for his reaction.

There is no way that he can conceal his true feelings. Whether he is shocked by the extent of the scars, or relieved that they aren't as bad as he had expected, his reaction will show on his face. The best way to handle the situation is for him to take her into his arms and hold her very close, thus reassuring her that together they can handle it. Husband and wife need each other's love and support to face the operation's effects on their lives.

Invariably, the woman will ask her husband if he can still find her attractive with only one breast. This is the time that he should tell her all the reasons why he loves her. He should emphasize that physical appearance is not nearly as important as personality and attitude. "But I'm just not like that!" some men protest. "If I started talking about all that stuff now, she'd be convinced that I've gone crazy!" Chances are she'd think he was the most beautiful man in the world. But if he really can't muster up the courage to tell her seriously, then he can reassure her through humor. For example, he could say, "Of course I think you're attractive. After all, you've still got your big toes and they're the real reason I fell in love with you." She'll get the message.

The single, most effective way that a husband can reassure his wife of his love is through sexual intercourse. Ideally, sexual relations should be resumed the very day she returns home from the hospital. But some women are afraid to go ahead with sexual intercourse because they are still suffering intense pain, or because they fear they will injure themselves in the process. The husband must be very careful to determine whether his wife's refusal of his advances stems from legitimate pain, or a fear that she will be rejected once the scars are exposed. Perhaps the best plan is to start out with kissing and gentle caressing to see how the woman will react. If she responds passionately, then sexual relations should follow without delay. If the woman prefers not to have sexual intercourse, then her wishes should be respected. This means that the husband does not stomp out of the room because his desires were not satisfied; instead, he expresses his understanding for her feelings and agrees to settle for less strenuous expressions of affection. But he should not wait for her to make the first move. He should keep up the kissing and caressing each day until his wife feels well enough to respond to his advances. And, by the way, if the couple has always made love with the lights on, they should continue to do so. A sudden change to darkness would be symbolic of rejection.

While his wife dresses, the husband often leaves the room out of consideration for his wife's feelings. This is exactly the *wrong* thing to do. Instead of decreasing his wife's anxiety, his leaving accomplishes just the opposite: she feels that her husband can't bear to look at her, and she has no one with her to share her pain when she looks in the mirror. The husband should make a point of remaining in the room if he did so previous to the surgery; he should look at her body in exactly the same way he always has. His actions reassure her that he is still attracted to her.

Unfortunately, some husbands find it impossible to offer their wives support and encouragement because they are themselves psychologically damaged by the mastectomy. A man who finds himself in this position needs professional help. Usually his problems can be traced back to his fear that his wife will die and leave him alone, unable to cope with his

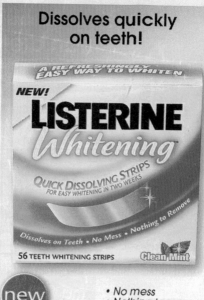
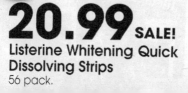

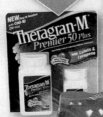
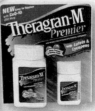

family responsibilities. This man should remember that the odds are in his wife's favor; if her cancer was caught early and treated properly, the chances are that she won't have a recurrence or a metastasis.

Of course, if the wife's cancer was already in an advanced state when it was discovered, her chances are not as encouraging. But in this case, the husband should remember that life offers none of us a guarantee that our loved ones will be alive tomorrow. Who knows? The wife with advanced breast cancer could even outlive her husband.

But once the husband knows that his wife is going to die, he can react two ways. He can withdraw from his emotional involvement with her so that perhaps it won't hurt as much when she dies, or he can draw nearer his wife and enjoy their remaining years together as fully as possible. Most husbands do want to draw emotionally closer to their wives, but they just don't know how. For these men, professional help is a must. The gynecologist or surgeon who treated the wife can assist the husband in finding the right help at the right price. There are many mental health clinics that offer free psychological counseling, and almost all churches have clergy who are trained to help, too.

In some ways having a mastectomy is like having a new baby in the house. It can draw a loving couple closer together or it can drive an unhappily married couple farther apart. A lot of time, energy, and love is required to make it through the anxious times. If either of the people involved doesn't feel that their future together is worth the extra effort, then the marriage is doomed.

When this is the case, it is mutually self-destructive to remain together. A husband who stays with his wife only because he'd feel guilty leaving her now that she's had a mastectomy, can't be much of a husband; sooner or later he's bound to stray and that is the ultimate rejection. A wife who remains with her husband only because she's afraid that she could never attract another man can't be much of a wife; she's denying herself a chance for real happiness. There are plenty of women who have met and married after losing one or both breasts to cancer. Their loving husbands know that breasts are not a prime factor in picking out a wife.

When there seems to be no solution to the failing marriage's problems, the best therapy for both individuals may be divorce. The husband and wife, with the aid of a professional marriage counselor or their minister, should discuss their real reasons for divorce. It is all too easy to blame the whole mess on the mastectomy. But in fact, the mastectomy serves only as a catalyst in the break-up. In the face of post-surgical stresses, the pre-existing anxieties the couple harbored came to the surface, and made adjustment impossible. The cancer didn't ruin the marriage—the people did.

The woman who has had a mastectomy, and has subsequently suffered through the agonies of a divorce, needs her friends and family more than ever. She needs their support not only for adapting to her altered appearance, but also for finding a new identity as a single person. The best way to help her realize this new identity is to praise her for taking on new responsibilities and handling them well. The one thing she does not need is so-called "constructive criticism." Criticism in the wake of a mastectomy and divorce is tantamount to saying "You dummy! Not only can't you control your own body, you can't even run your own life!"

Any woman who has been married for years and suddenly finds herself single again will make mistakes before things start going well. Give her time. Talk with her about what she's doing, but let her draw her own conclusions. The lessons she learns from her mistakes will help her adjust better to her mastectomy, and aid her in establishing her single-person identity.

One day it will suddenly be clear to her that none of us has total control over our life; we simply do the best we can with what we've got. Let her do the best she can, but be sure to tell her what a great deal she's got.

To do this, think about the old song lyric "You gotta accentuate the positive and eliminate the negative." While you cannot eliminate the fact that she now has only one breast, you don't have to dwell on it. Instead, tell her how many friends she has who will support her in any endeavor *and then support her.* Tell her she can always depend on you for a sounding board for her ideas and plans *and then listen to her.* Emphasize her many talents *and then praise her for using them constructively.* Your follow-up of each positive factor is necessary to reinforce the value she places on these factors herself.

Chapter Fourteen

AND WHAT OF OUR DAUGHTERS AND GRANDDAUGHTERS?

Within ten years the standard treatment for breast cancer may change drastically. The radical and modified radical mastectomies that are the standard treatment today may be abandoned in favor of less mutilating operations. By 1980, we'll be able to compare those ten-year survival statistics that most doctors consider to be really significant. If the simpler operations are proved to be equally effective, the experimental procedures of today will become the preferred treatment for women with early breast cancer. Increased availability of breast cancer screening programs should mean that breast cancers will be caught early.

Recent studies of radioactive implants of Iridium 192 have shown the implants to be at least as effective as surgery for treating localized early and advanced breast cancers. In this procedure, plastic tubes containing the radioactive substance are positioned inside the breast tumor and left in place for three to five days. The breast is *not* removed. Although the technique has been known for almost twenty years, it is just now being considered as a substitute for the traditional radiation treatments that take up to eight weeks of daily treatments to be effective.

When you consider that the survival rates for surgically treated breast cancers have not changed in almost one hundred years, despite advances in operating techniques, it seems obvious that surgery is not the ideal treatment. Chemotherapy, now in its infancy, may turn out to be that ideal treatment. We already know that the earliest chemotherapy treatments administered to breast cancer patients were 20% effective in preventing recurrences and metastases after radical mastectomy. Surely that effectiveness can be improved. The 50-50 chance that mastectomy offers, to women whose lymph nodes are already cancerous at the time of surgery, is totally unacceptable. The role of chemotherapy in conjunction with mastectomy, or radiation implants, should be expanded and improved.

But in the meantime, those women who have already had mastectomies now have some hope for reconstruction (rebuilding). If the skin covering the chest is in good condition (and usually this means that no radiation treatments have been given), a skin flap can be used to cover a silicone implant. These implants are perfectly legal and are much safer than silicone injections. In fact, the only danger with a silicone implant is that the shadows it casts on X ray film will block a tiny recurrence, which will then remain undetected and develop into a full-blown tumor. This is why most surgeons prefer to wait five to ten years after the original surgery to start reconstruction. With present techniques the reconstructed breast only approximates the appearance of a normal breast. There is no nipple unless you are willing to give up either your navel or some tissue from your genital area to have one made. The reconstruction procedure is very expensive and usually requires a series of hospitalizations. Very few insurance companies will cover even a portion of the expenses since they consider breast reconstruction to be medically unnecessary, cosmetic surgery.

Some surgeons have been experimenting with a procedure called subcutaneous mastectomy with immediate reconstruction. The idea is to make an incision beneath the breast in the skin fold and scoop out the breast tissue through this opening. The skin, nipple, and some supportive tissue is left intact. A silicone implant is then inserted through the incision and the wound is closed. With the scar hidden in the skin fold, no one would ever suspect that the woman has had a mastectomy. This procedure works out very well for women who want their breasts removed because of recurrent benign breast disease. But the procedure is not advisable for women with breast cancer because of the extremely high probability that the milk ducts, and therefore the nipple, have already been invaded by cancer cells.

Scientists are optimistic that breast cancer will someday be treated nonsurgically and possibly will even be preventable. As soon as the genetic (hereditary) controls of breast cancer are clearly defined, chromosome tests could easily determine which newborn girls are highly susceptible to breast cancer. Once these girls are identified, preventive measures could be applied. Mother Nature's most effective protection against breast cancer is early pregnancy. Girls who are high risk could arrange to have a baby very early in life, preferably before the age of twenty. If having a child at this age wouldn't be appropriate for her (for religious or other reasons), perhaps she could resort to immunotherapy, or medicines that would activate her body's immune response to fight off any immature cancer cells, or cancer cell precursors which might be forming. At the very least, these girls could be advised not to take birth control pills, but to rely on some other form of contraception.

As researchers identify the specific environmental and dietary factors that contribute significantly to cancer growth, prevention becomes possible through the elimination of carcinogens (cancer-causing chemicals) from the environment and from food substances. Of course this clean-up campaign would take many years, possibly decades, to achieve its goal. Meanwhile some preventive vaccine would have to be offered through mass-immunization programs to women who live in high-risk areas.

Researchers may actually be on their way to developing a vaccine that will prevent breast cancer. Their experiments with mice that have breast cancer have shown that blood serum from women with certain types of breast cancers can be used as a very effective treatment. If it's possible to neutralize mouse breast cancers with serum from humans with breast cancer, then why not the opposite? The blood serum from some mice with breast cancer may cure or even prevent some human breast cancers.

Research is a long, slow process. Sometimes it seems as if breast cancer will never be brought under control, especially when you consider that the treatment has remained basically unchanged for almost a hundred years. But we *will* see definitive statistics on surgical techniques within five to ten years; and we *may* see development of an effective vaccine within our lifetimes. With current improvements in early diagnosis of breast cancers, it is possible that our daughters will never experience the disfigurement of radical mastectomy. It's even possible that our granddaughters will never even know what it's like to fear breast cancer.

Chapter Fifteen

FAST SOURCES OF BREAST CANCER INFORMATION AND BREAST CANCER SCREENING CLINICS

Breast Cancer Hotline: (301) 897-8808

Operated by The Breast Cancer Advisory Service
P.O. Box 422
Kensington, Maryland 20795

Reach to Recovery:
  Sponsored by the American Cancer Society.
Your local unit is listed in the white pages of your telephone book under "American Cancer Society." *Or,* you can write to the national headquarters at this address: American Cancer Society
            777 Third Avenue
            New York, N.Y. 10017

The following breast cancer screening clinics are funded jointly by the American Cancer Society and the National Cancer Institute to demonstrate the value of early detection of occult breast cancers. In accordance with this purpose, the examinations are available only to women who do *not* have any symptoms of breast cancer. If you already have a breast lump, you do not qualify for these programs. But if you are merely looking for a way to get your annual breast examination, and your breasts appear to be normal, you may wish to call one of these centers. New screening clinics may be opening up closer to where you live. To find out if there is one, contact your nearest branch of the American Cancer Society.

Arizona   Arizona Medical Center
Tucson, Arizona 85724
(602) 882-7401 or 7402

California   John Wesley Hospital
Los Angeles, California 90033
(213) 748-5379

Samuel Merritt Hospital
Breast Screening Center
384 34th Street
Oakland, California 94609
(415) 658-8525

Delaware   Wilmington General Hospital
Chestnut and Broom Streets
Wilmington, Delaware 19899
(302) 428-4815

District of Columbia Georgetown University
Medical School
3800 Reservoir Road, N.W.
Washington, D.C. 20007
(202) 625-2183

Florida St. Vincent's Medical Center
Barrs Street and St. Johns Avenue
Jacksonville, Florida 32204
(904) 389-7751, Ext. 8491 or 8492

Georgia Georgia Baptist Hospital
340 Boulevard N.E.
Atlanta, Georgia 30312
(404) 525-7861

Hawaii Pacific Health Research Institute, Inc.
Alexander Young Building, Suite 545
Hotel and Bishop Streets
Honolulu, Hawaii 96813
(808) 524-4337

Idaho Mountain States Tumor Institute
215 Avenue B
Boise, Idaho 83702
(208) 345-3590

Iowa Iowa Lutheran Hospital
University at Penn
Des Moines, Iowa 50316
(515) 283-5678

Kansas University of Kansas Medical Center
Rainbow Boulevard at 39th Street
Kansas City, Kansas 66103
(913) 342-1338

Kentucky University of Louisville School of
Medicine
601 S. Floyd Street
Louisville, Kentucky 40402
(502) 583-2894

Michigan University of Michigan Medical Center
396 W. Washington Street
Ann Arbor, Michigan 48103
(313) 763-0056

Missouri Cancer Research Center
Business Loop, 70th and Garth Avenue
Columbia, Missouri 65201
(314) 443-2216

New Jersey College of Medicine and Dentistry of
New Jersey
15 S. 9th Street
Newark, New Jersey 07107
(201) 484-9221

New York Guttman Institute
200 Madison Avenue at 35th Street
New York, New York 10016
(212) 689-9797

North Carolina Duke University Medical Center
3040 Erwin Road
Durham, North Carolina 27705
(919) 286-7943 or 383-1060

Ohio University of Cincinnati Medical Center
Eden and Bethesda Avenues
Cincinnati, Ohio 45229
(513) 872-5331

Oklahoma Oklahoma Medical Research
Foundation
800 N.E. 8th Street
Oklahoma City, Oklahoma 73190
(405) 235-8331, ext. 241

Oregon Breast Cancer Screening Project
2222 N.W. Lovejoy
Portland, Oregon 97210
(503) 229-7292

Pennsylvania Temple University
3401 N. Broad Street
Philadelphia, Pennsylvania 19140
(215) 221-3832

University of Pittsburgh School
of Medicine
The Falk Clinic
3601 Fifth Avenue
Pittsburgh, Pennsylvania 15213
(412) 624-3336

Rhode Island Rhode Island Hospital
Rhode Island Department of Health
Eddy Street
Providence, Rhode Island 02908
(401) 831-6970

Tennessee Vanderbilt University School of
Medicine
Nashville, Tennessee 37322
(615) 322-2501

Texas St. Joseph's Hospital
1919 La Branch
Houston, Texas 77002
(713) 225-3131, ext. 301

Washington Virginia Mason Medical Center
911 Seneca Street
Seattle, Washington 98101
(206) 624-1144

Wisconsin Medical College of Wisconsin
8700 W. Wisconsin Avenue
Milwaukee, Wisconsin 53236
(414) 257-5200

Chapter Sixteen

DIRECTORY OF BREAST FORM MANUFACTURERS

You can write to the manufacturers listed in this directory to get copies of their brochures and the names of distributors near your home. In general, breast prostheses are available in corset shops, department store lingerie and foundation departments, and medical supply stores. Department stores are usually the least expensive and medical supply stores the most expensive.

Comparison shopping for a breast form is important for more than just pricing. You may find that one store's fitter is more knowledgeable than the others, or that one store charges a fitting fee and another does not.

There are many types of breast forms, as the following directory will show. The prices vary from as low as $6.00 to as high as $175, depending on the style you choose. The less-expensive models are air- and liquid-filled styles which, because of their light weight, are particularly good for small-breasted women or for women whose incisions are still tender. The silicone gel models, which are in the intermediate price range, are good for medium- to full-breasted women; the added weight of the silicone gel helps to balance the weight of the natural breast and thus can improve the posture by helping to keep the shoulders level. The most expensive prostheses are specially made reproductions of the remaining breast—they are colored to match your natural skin color and even have an areola and nipple. Aesthetic appeal is the only real advantage to these breast forms.

A very real inequity of our medical system surrounds the purchase of the breast prosthesis. Most insurance companies will pay for only the first breast form you buy, and even then they will often pay for only part of the cost; for some reason, insurance companies think that breast forms are cosmetic appliances that are not really necessary. This system encourages women to buy the most expensive form they can get, which is totally wrong medically. A woman who has just recently undergone mastectomy needs a very lightweight form (such as an air- or liquid-filled style); a very heavy form—the most expensive—will only aggravate the wound.

When shopping for your first prosthesis, try to arrange for your Reach to Recovery volunteer to accompany you. You can profit from her experience.

Unweighted and Weighted Rubber Prostheses

Trademark	Manufacturer	Price	Comments
Lové	Lové 7494 Santa Monica Blvd. Hollywood, Calif. 90046	$20 and up	Good for thin, small-breasted women and as temporary prosthesis after the lounger, and before heavily weighted permanent prosthesis. Weight is adjustable.
Silveco	Silveco Products, Inc. 2502 Milwaukee Avenue Chicago, Ill. 60647	$6 and up	Good for thin, small-breasted women and as temporary prosthesis after the lounger, and before heavily weighted permanent prosthesis.

Air-Filled Plastic Prostheses

Trademark	Manufacturer	Price	Comments
Ideal Form	Ideal-Form, Inc. P.O. Box 777 Orange, Conn. 06477	$4 and up	Suitable for thin, small-breasted women. Cannot be worn in airplanes that are not pressurized.* Provides underarm fullness.
Atco	Atco Surgical Supports 450 Portage Trail Cuyahoga Falls, Ohio 44222	$4.50	Suitable for thin, small-breasted women. Cannot be worn in airplanes that are not pressurized.* Provides underarm fullness.
Tres-Secrete	Camp International P.O. Box 89 Jackson, Mich. 49204	$8.50 to $10.50	Suitable for thin, small-breasted women. Cannot be worn in airplanes that are not pressurized.* Very good for woman who has had both breasts removed.

*If worn in an unpressurized airplane, the air inside the prosthesis will expand and cause the prosthesis to explode.

Air-and-Fluid-Filled Prostheses

Trademark	Manufacturer	Price	Comments
Confidante	Spencer Medical Division Berger Brothers Company 135 Derby Avenue New Haven, Conn. 06507	$40	Size is adjustable by inflating or deflating air part. Available through J.C. Penney catalog.
Identical Form	Identical Form 17 W. 60th Street New York, N.Y. 10023	$25	Natural weight. Can be worn with regular bra. May be uncomfortable in hot weather. Tends to leak.
Restoration	Restoration P.O. Box 1541 Fairfield, Conn. 06430	$39	Not widely used.

Liquid-Filled Prostheses

Trademark	Manufacturer	Price	Comments
Mastectomy Form	Mastectomy Form R3 B 64S Town East Monroe, La. 71201	$30 and up	Available in simple and radical models.
Naturelles	Camp International P.O. Box 89 Jackson, Miss. 49204	$6.50	Designed for women who have had partial mastectomies, either unilateral or bilateral.
Brest Form	Atco Surgical Supports 450 Portage Trail Cuyahoga Falls, Ohio 44222	$35 and up	Can be ordered through Sears and Montgomery Ward catalogs. Fills hollows.
Tru-Life	Camp International P.O. Box 89 Jackson, Mich. 49204	$40	Alters to accommodate weight changes. Soft, pliable, natural-looking. Very heavily weighted. Leaks when punctured. Must be worn with special bra that costs $12.50 and up, or regular bra can be modified.

Silicone Gel-Filled Prostheses

Trademark	Manufacturer	Price	Comments
Companion	Airway Surgical Co Erie Avenue Cincinnati, Ohio 45209	$90 and up	Doesn't slip. Natural look, weight, and feel. Can be worn with regular bra. Can be uncomfortable in hot weather.
La Meme	Camp International, Inc. P.O. Box 89 Jackson, Mich. 49204	$80 and up	Natural look, weight, and feel.
Active	Stryker Corp. 420 Alcott Street Kalamazoo. Mich. 49001	$75 and up	Currently being redesigned.

Combination Prostheses

Trademark	Manufacturer	Price	Comments
Jodee	Jodee, Inc. 200 Madison Ave. New York, N.Y. 10016	$45 and up	Natural look and feel. Adjusts to weight changes. Fills hollows. Must be worn with special bra that costs $15 and up.

Custom-Made Prostheses

Trademark	Manufacturer	Price	Comments
Match Mate	Dr. Eugene L. Harris 1203 N. Euclid Anaheim, Calif. 92801	$175 and up	Exact duplication of remaining breast made by molded impression. Not widely available.
Perfect Mate	Ruth Merzon 233 W. 77th Street New York, N.Y. 10024	$50 and up	Not widely available.

Glossary

ABDOMEN: Belly.

ADJUNCTIVE THERAPY: Treatment given in addition to some other treatment, e.g. radiation therapy is "adjunctive" to simple mastectomy.

ADRENAL GLANDS: A pair of glands located just on top of the kidneys.

ADRENALECTOMY: Surgical removal of the adrenal glands.

ADRENAL STERIODS: Hormones produced by the interior parts of the adrenal glands; after menopause, these hormones are converted into estrogens through biochemical transformation.

AMBULATION: Walking.

ANDROGENS: The so-called "male" hormones which, in fact, are normally present in both males and females.

ANESTHESIA: Loss of feeling.

ANESTHETIC: Substance used to induce a state of anesthesia.

ANESTHESIOLOGIST: Doctor whose medical specialty is the administration of anesthetics and monitoring of body functions during surgery.

AREOLA: The dark skin surrounding the nipple of the breast.

ANTIBODY: When foreign or alien substances, such as bacteria, enter the body, the body must "decide" whether it's good for you or harmful. If harmful, the body manufactures an antibody which works together with white blood cells to fight off the bad substance.

ANTIGEN: The outside surface of the invading bacteria by which the body recognizes and decides whether or not it belongs in your body.

ANXIETY: Feeling of apprehension or uncertainty.

ARTERIOSCLEROSIS: A disease marked by fatty deposits in the arteries.

ASPIRATION BIOPSY: Insertion of a long, thin hypodermic needle into a suspected tumor in order to retrieve cells for miscroscopic examination.

AUTOPSY: Examination of a body after death in order to determine the cause of death.

BACTERIA: Microscopic disease-carrying organisms.

BENIGN: Not cancerous.

BILATERAL: Both sides.

BILIARY HORMONES: Hormones in the bile, secreted by the liver.

BIOFEEDBACK: Mental control over bodily functions.

BIOPSY: Process of obtaining tissue samples for microscopic examination.

BLOOD PRESSURE: The pressure that the blood exerts on the walls of the arteries.

BLOOD SERUM: The liquid portion of the blood.

BLOOD VESSEL: An artery or a vein: the canals through which the blood flows as it travels throughout the body.

BOARDS: Examinations that a doctor must pass before he is considered a specialist.

BOARD CERTIFIED: Referring to a doctor who has passed the boards.

BREAST: The mammary gland, peculiar to mammals, which is responsible for producing milk for nourishing the young.

BREASTBONE: The sternum. The bone situated immediately under the skin in the middle of the chest.

BREAST CANCER SCREENING CLINIC: A clinic which provides free or low-cost breast examinations, including thermography, mammography, and/or xerography.

BREAST FORM: A breast prosthesis, or artificial breast, for use after mastectomy.

BROAD SPECTRUM ANTIBIOTIC: A drug designed to kill a wide variety of bacteria as opposed to one that kills only a very specific bacterium, Tetracycline is a broad-spectrum antibiotic.

CANCER: A tumor that is usually associated with formation of secondary tumors or metastases.

CARCINOGEN: A substance that causes cancer.

CARCINOGENIC: Cancer-causing.

CELL: The entire body is made from cells. The bloodstream, muscles, organs, etc., are many cells grouped together.

CERVIX: The entrance to the uterus or womb.

CHEMOTHERAPY: Treatment of disease by administration of drugs.

CHEST WALL: The rib cage and the muscles covering it.

CHROMOSOME: Microscopic structures that contain the genes, the blueprints of all hereditary traits.

CHRONIC: Continuing over a long period of time.

COMPLICATION: A new disease or condition that aggravates the existing disease, or makes recovery after surgery more difficult.

CONFLICT: A clash of two opposing viewpoints held by one person.

CONSENT FOR SURGERY: The written form that gives the surgeon permission to go ahead with the agreed-upon operation.

CORSETIERE: Corset shop.

CONSULTATION: The deliberation of two or more doctors in an effort to make a diagnosis or select appropriate therapy.

CONTRACEPTION: Prevention of pregnancy.

CYST: A fluid filled sac-like structure that appears as a breast lump.

CYSTIC FIBROSIS: A hereditary, chronic disease of the lungs and pancreas characterized by inability to digest foods and difficulty in breathing.

DEHYDRATED: Dried up; a state of severe water loss.

DEPENDENCE/INDEPENDENCE CONFLICT: Inner clash of desire to be self-sufficient and desire to be taken care of.

DEPRESSION: Emotional dejection, often similar to a "bad mood."

DIAGNOSIS: Identification of a specific disease as the cause of a person's illness.

DOCTOR-PATIENT RELATIONSHIP: Feeling of mutual trust between a patient and his doctor.

DRAINAGE TUBE: Plastic, flexible tubes that, connected with a vacuum pump, drain excess fluids away from the surgical wound site.

ECZEMA: A disease which causes the skin to look crusty and scaly.

EDEMA: Swelling due to retained fluids.

EGG: The microscopic cell released from the ovary which, when fertilized by the male sperm, eventually becomes a baby.

ELECTROCARDIOGRAM: A test which measures the electrical currents produced when the heart beats.

EMERGENCY ROOM: That portion of the hospital which is designed to handle medical and surgical cases that must be treated immediately.

ENZYME: A chemical that promotes biochemical transformation of one substance into another.

EROGENOUS ZONE: Any area of the body that,

when caressed, produces sexual arousal.

ESTRADIOL: An estrogen with carcinogenic potential.

ESTRIOL: An estrogen that counteracts the carcinogenic potential of estradiol and estrone.

ESTRONE: An estrogen with carcinogenic potential.

ESTROGENS: The so-called "female" hormones that are, in fact, found in both males and females.

EXTENDED RADICAL MASTECTOMY: Surgical removal of the breast, the lymph nodes of the outer chest wall, armpit, and under the breastbone, and the pectoral muscles.

FALSE-NEGATIVE: A breast cancer that is called benign on the basis of clinical and X-ray findings, but which turns out to be malignant at biopsy.

FALSE-POSITIVE: A breast cancer that is called malignant on the basis of clinical and X-ray findings, but which turns out to be benign at biopsy.

FAMILY DOCTOR: The doctor seen regularly for physical examinations and illnesses.

FATS: Fatty substances consumed in the diet in such forms as meats, dairy products, and shellfish.

FIBROADENOMA: A fibrous tumor that appears as a breast lump, particularly common in young women.

FIBROCYSTIC DISEASE OF THE BREAST: Formation of fibrous tumors and cysts that appear as lumps in the breast, particularly common in middle-aged women.

FIBROUS: Made up of fibers.

FIVE-YEAR SURVIVAL RATES: The percentage of women still alive five years after cancer surgery.

FLUOROSCOPY: A kind of X-ray machine that enables the doctor to see inside his patient's body by means of a special screen.

FOREIGN: Not natural to the body. That is, food is "foreign" as is medicine; but so are germs (bacteria).

FOREPLAY: Sexual contact that precedes intercourse.

FROZEN SECTION: The preliminary biopsy examination performed on a thin piece of tissue that is quick-frozen, but not stained.

FULL-TERM PREGNANCY: A pregnancy of nine months duration; a pregnancy that is not interrupted by abortion, miscarriage, or premature birth of the infant.

GENERAL ANESTHESIA: Loss of consciousness and ability to feel pain.

GENETIC: Inherited from the mother and father through the egg and sperm, respectively.

GENITAL: Pertaining to the reproductive organs.

GLAND: An organ that produces a specific product or secretion.

GYNECOLOGIST: A doctor whose specialty is treating the diseases that are unique to women.

HALSTED RADICAL MASTECTOMY: The surgical removal of the breast, pectoral muscles, and the lymph nodes of the outer chest wall and armpit, as described by Halsted in 1894.

HEMATOMA: A small puddle of blood that has escaped into the body tissues from the blood vessels as a result of injury.

HEREDITY: The inheritance of traits or diseases from one's parents or ancestors.

HIGH-RISK GROUP: Those women who are statistically most likely to develop breast cancer.

HOLLOWS: Indentations left in the upper chest after removal of the pectoral muscles in radical mastectomy.

HORMONE: A substance produced by a gland.

HORMONE DEPENDENT: Most cancers can exist without the presence of hormones. Those which need hormones in order to grow are called hormone dependent.

HORMONE THERAPY: Alteration of the natural hormone balance in order to control the growth of hormone-dependent cancers.

HOSTILITY: Feelings of hatred or opposition.

HYPERTENSION: High blood pressure.

HYPERCALCEMIA: An excess of calcium in the blood.

HYPOPHYSECTOMY: Surgical removal of the pituitary gland.

HYPOTHYROIDISM: Deficiency in thyroid function.

HYSTERECTOMY: Surgical removal of the uterus.

IMMUNE: Protected against a disease.

IMMUNE RESPONSE: The process by which the body fights off disease-carrying organisms that invade the body.

IMMUNOLOGICAL: Pertaining to the immune

response.

INFANT MORTALITY RATE: The percentage of all babies that are born dead or die shortly after birth.

IMMUNIZATION: Administration of a vaccine that renders the patient immune to a specific disease.

IMMUNOTHERAPY: Administration of medicines that stimulate the immune response.

INFORMED CONSENT: Consent for a procedure by a patient who understands exactly what the doctor will do, what kind of risk it involves, and the possible adverse or side effects.

INHALATION ANESTHESIC: Anesthesic that is administered in a gaseous form that is breathed by the patient.

INSOMNIA: Inability to sleep.

INTRAVENOUS: Directly into a blood vein.

IRRADIATION: Treatment with X rays.

KLINEFELTER'S SYNDROME: An inherited chromosomal abnormality that affects men.

LISTLESSNESS: Disinterest, general fatigue.

LOCAL ANESTHESIA: Loss of ability to feel pain in only a portion of the body and without loss of consciousness.

LOCALIZED TUMOR: A tumor that is well confined to a small area of the body, as opposed to a tumor that has spread to the normal tissue surrounding it (called an invasive tumor).

LOUNGER: Temporary breast prosthesis that is lightweight and intended to be worn within a few days after mastectomy.

LUMPECTOMY: Partial mastectomy.

LYMPH: Combination of excess fluids, white blood cells, and dead cells.

LYMPH CHANNEL: Vessel which carries lymph toward the heart.

LYMPH NODE: Glandlike structure that filters bacteria and other contaminants that would otherwise be absorbed into the lymph channels.

LYMPHATIC SYSTEM: Network of lymph nodes and lymph channels throughout the body.

MALIGNANCY: A cancer.

MALIGNANT: Cancerous.

MAMMOGRAPHY: The process for an X ray of the breast.

MAMMOGRAM: X-ray film made through mammography process.

MARRIAGE COUNSELOR: Professional person who advises and assists husbands and wives in matters related to their marriage. Usually this person holds a degree in psychology or social work.

MASOCHISTIC: Self-punishing. Describes someone who enjoys physical or mental suffering.

MASTECTOMY: Surgical removal of all or part of the breast, sometimes accompanied by removal of surrounding tissue or muscle. See the specific kinds of mastectomies for further information.

MASTITIS: Infection of the breast.

MASTURBATION: Auto-eroticism; stimulation of oneself to orgasm.

MATERNAL DEATH RATE: The percentage of mothers who die during delivery of a baby, or shortly thereafter due to complications of the delivery itself.

MEDICAID: A government program of health insurance for persons of all ages whose incomes are limited.

MEDICAL HISTORY: A thorough and complete record of a patient's past illnesses, along with any inheritable diseases that have occurred among his family.

MEDICARE: A federal program of health insurance for people over 65 years of age.

MENARCHE: The onset of menstruation.

MENOPAUSE: The cessation of menstruation.

MENSTRUAL CYCLE: Individual pattern of menstruation; i.e., some women get their period every 28 days, others every 30 days, etc.

MENSTRUATION: The cyclic uterine bleeding which normally occurs about every 28 days in the absence of pregnancy.

METABOLIZE: How the body changes one substance into another; for example, how the foods we eat are converted into energy.

METASTASIS: To *metastasize* is to spread from one part of the body to anther. The metastasis is the actual tumor which forms at the new site.

MICROSCOPE: An instrument used to see things that are so small they cannot be seen by the naked eye.

MILK DUCT: Channel through which breast milk passes to the nipple.

MODIFIED RADICAL MASTECTOMY: Surgical removal of the breast and the lymph nodes of the outer chest wall, base of the neck, and armpit.

MOLYBDENUM TUBE: A special kind of tube

used to make X-ray machines effective for use as mammography units.

MYASTHENIA GRAVIS: Disease characterized by progressive exhaustion of the muscles, especially the muscles of the face and neck.

NAVEL: Belly button.

NEUROTIC: A person whose emotions dominate reason.

NIPPLE: The point of the breast through which milk passes as a baby sucks on the breast.

NITRITES: Carcinogenic chemicals commonly used to preserve some meats and cheeses.

OCCULT CANCER: A cancer that is not evident upon physical examination.

ONCOLOGIST: A specialist in internal medicine whose subspecialty is the treatment of cancers.

OOPHORECTOMY: Ovariectomy.

ORGASM: The physical and emotional sensation experienced at the height of sexual intercourse or masturbation.

OUTPATIENT DEPARTMENT: That part of a hospital designed to care for patients who are not sick enough to be admitted as regular patients, and who are not required to stay in bed.

OVARIECTOMY: Surgical removal of the ovaries.

OVARY: The female sexual gland in which the egg is formed; the main source of estrogens before menopause.

PALPABLE: Detectable when gently prodded or touched.

PALPATE: Gently prod and push in order to feel the contours of underlying structures.

PAP SMEAR: Light scraping of the cervix in order

to obtain cells for microscopic study; the test for cancer of the cervix.

PAPILLOMA: Nipple discharge.

PARTIAL MASTECTOMY: Surgical removal of a breast cancer and a wedge of the surrounding tissue. Lumpectomy.

PATHOLOGIST: The doctor whose specialty is studying the structural and functional changes of tissues and organs as the result of disease.

PECTORALIS MUSCLES: The muscles covering the chest wall, specifically the pectoralis major and pectoralis minor.

PECTORALS: The pectoralis muscles.

PELVIC EXAMINATION: Internal examination of the female reproductive organs.

PERSONALITY: Traits that make a person a unique human being, different from all others.

PITUITARY GLAND: A tiny gland located at the base of the brain; specifically, the *hypophysis cerebri.*

POST-OPERATIVE: After an operation.

POST-SURGICAL: After surgery.

PRIMARY TUMOR: The original cancer as opposed to a secondary tumor or metastasis.

PROLACTIN: The hormone which, in pregnant women, stimulates milk production.

PROSTHESIS: An artificial breast designed to be worn after mastectomy.

PSYCHIATRIST: A doctor whose specialty is treatment of mental and emotional disorders.

PSYCHOLOGIST: A person (not a doctor of medicine) who holds a degree in psychology and treats emotional problems. He cannot prescribe drug therapies such as tranquilizers, antidepressants, etc., as can the psychiatrist.

PSYCHOTHERAPY: Treatment of emotional disorders by attempting to remove the cause of the disorder.

PULSE: Expansion and contraction of an artery as can be felt at the inner aspect of the wrist or in the neck just below the jaw.

RADIATION: Treatment by X rays or radioactive implants.

RADIATION FIELD: That area exposed to irradiation during radiation therapy.

RADIATION THERAPY: Irradiation of a tumor in order to cause tumor shrinkage or to kill beginning cancer cells.

RADICAL MASTECTOMY: see Halsted radical mastectomy.

RADIATION IMPLANT: Plastic tubes filled with radioactive material that are inserted directly into a cancer in an effort to cause tumor shrinkage or to kill cancer cells.

RADIOACTIVE IMPLANT: see radiation implant.

RADIOLOGIST: A doctor whose speciality is the diagnosis and treatment of disease with the aid of X rays, radioactive substances, and high-frequency sound waves.

REACH TO RECOVERY: A program sponsored by the American Cancer Society to help women who have had mastectomies.

RECONSTRUCTION: Rebuilding of a missing part through plastic surgery.

RECOVERY ROOM: The room where surgical

patients stay after their operations until they have recovered from the effect of anesthetic.

RECTUM: The end of the digestive system where solid waste products are stored until eliminated.

RECURRENCE: Return of cancer at its original site.

REMISSION: Period in which symptoms of a disease diminish or disappear temporarily.

RESERPINE: A drug used to treat high blood pressure.

RESIDENCY: A specialty training program requiring two or more years of specialized work after graduation from medical school.

RESIDENT: A doctor who is currently doing his residency.

RIB CAGE: The basketlike structure formed by the ribs around the lungs.

SCAN: A diagnostic examination in which radioactive materials are injected into the bloodstream and followed as they course through the body and are eventually absorbed.

SELF: Philosophically, that portion of the mind which knows, reflects, suffers, desires, etc., as opposed to that which is known, remembered, etc.; i.e., one's emotions rather than memory or logic.

SELF-CONCEPT: One's own image of what constitutes the real self, or how a person sees himself—not what others see.

SELF-EXAMINATION: Examination of her own breasts by the concerned woman.

SELF-REALIZATION: Fulfillment of one's potential capacities; to succeed in one's goals.

SEXUAL INTERCOURSE: Physical union of male and female; lovemaking.

SIBLING: Brother or sister.

SIDE EFFECT: An effect of a drug that is in addition to its intended effect.

SILICONE IMPLANT: A breast-shaped plastic bag filled with silicone gel, designed to be placed under the skin to simulate a real breast.

SILICONE INJECTIONS: The injection of liquid silicone under the skin to enlarge the breasts or to fill in hollows in the chest or face. Silicone injections are illegal in the United States and are considered very dangerous.

SIMPLE MASTECTOMY: Surgical removal of the breast.

SPECIALIST: A doctor who has graduated from medical school, completed an approved residency, and passed his boards in a particular type of medicine.

SPECULUM: A plastic or metal device used to hold the vaginal walls apart during pelvic examination.

SPERM: The microscopic cells produced by the male which fertilize the female's egg to produce a baby.

STAGING: Systematic classification of cancers according to information obtained from physical examination, X rays, and pathological studies.

STAIN (A TISSUE SAMPLE): Process of dipping tissue samples into a series of dyes in order to stain microscopic structures for better visualization and examination.

STETHOSCOPE: The instrument used by doctors

to listen to heart and breathing sounds.

STITCH UP A WOUND: Sew up a wound with special surgical needles and sutures.

STRESS: Mental or emotional strain or tension.

SUBCUTANEOUS MASTECTOMY: Removal of breast tissue through an incision at the base of the breast, leaving the skin and nipple in place. Usually, silicone implants are slipped into the pocket to immediately reconstruct the breast.

SURGEON: A doctor whose specialty is surgery.

TEMPERATURE: Body heat as measured by a thermometer inserted in the mouth, in the rectum, or in the armpit.

THERMOGRAPHY: Measuring body heat by passing heat-sensitive devices over the skin to identify hot spots.

THYROID GLAND: A gland located over the trachea.

TOURNIQUET: Usually a rubber strip tied tightly around the upper arm to make the arm's blood vessels stand out in preparation for taking a blood sample.

TRACHEA: The top of the respiratory system; the windpipe.

TUMOR: Tissue which grows independently of its surroundings and serves no useful purpose.

UNILATERAL: On one side only.

URINE: The body's liquid wastes.

UTERUS: The womb; the part of the female body in which the baby develops.

VACCINE: A substance administered to make the recipient immune to a specific disease.

VACUUM PUMP: A small pump which, when

attached to surgical drainage tubes, sucks excess fluids out of the wound site.

VAGINA: The passageway from the uterus to the outside of the body; the birth canal.

VERTEBRA: One of the many small bones which make up the spine or backbone.

VIRGIN: A woman who has never had sexual intercourse.

VIRUS: A submicroscopic disease-causing organism.

WHITE BLOOD CELL: The type of blood cell responsible for "eating up" harmful bacteria, or foreign substances.

WIDE-BORE NEEDLE BIOPSY: Biopsy performed by inserting a large hollow needle into a breast tumor, and then passing a small surgical instrument through the needle to cut out a tissue sample.

WOUND: In surgery, the surgical incision.

XERORADIOGRAPHY: X ray of the breast using special Xerox techniques for development of the picture. Also called xerography.

X RAY: Use of invisible, high-energy waves to penetrate the human body and form images on photographic film.

BIBLIOGRAPHY

Ackerman, L.V., and del Regato, J.A. *Cancer: diagnosis, treatment, and prognosis.* 4th ed. St. Louis: Mosby, 1970.

"After mastectomy, finding the right prostheses." *Consumer Reports* pp. 652-4, November, 1975.

Aitken-Swan, J. and Paterson, R. "The cancer patient: delay in seeking advice." *British Medical Journal* 1:623, 1955.

"Animal study shows intriguing link between chronic stress and cancer." *Journal of the American Medical Association* 233:757-8, August 18, 1975.

Bacon C. L., et al. "A psychosomatic study of cancer

of the breast." *Psychosomatic Medicine* 14:453-60, 1952.

Bard, M. "The sequence of emotional reactions in radical mastectomy patients." *Public Health Reports* 67:1144-8, 1952.

Blum, R.H. *The commonsense guide to doctors, hospitals, and medical care.* New York: Macmillan, 1964.

Breast cancer: early and late. A collection of papers presented at the 13th annual clinical conference on cancer, 1968, at the University of Texas M.D. Anderson Hospital and Tumor Institute at Houston, Houston, Texas. Chicago: Yearbook, 1970.

"Breast cancer linked to 'pill' in state-UC study." Article in the *Los Angeles Times*, November 7, 1975.

Brinkley, D., and Haybittle, J.L. "Treatment of stage II carcinoma of the female breast." *Lancet* 2:291-5, 1966.

Cady, B. "Modern management of breast cancer. A point of view." *Archives of Surgery* 104:270-5, March, 1972.

Campion, R. *The invisible worm.* New York: Macmillan, 1972.

Cancer Facts and Figures. New York: American Cancer Society, 1975.

Charkes, N.D., et al. "Preoperative bone scans: use in women with early breast cancer." *Journal of the American Medical Association* 233:516-8, August 11, 1975.

Cobb B., et al. "Patient responsible delay of treatment in cancer: social psychological study." *Cancer*

7:920, 1954.

Cope, O. "Breast cancer: has the time come for a less mutilating treatment?" *Psychiatry in Medicine* 2:263-9, October, 1971.

Crile, G.H., Jr. "Results of simple mastectomy without irradiation in the treatment of operative stage I cancer of the breast." *Annals of Surgery* 168:330-4, 1968.

Crile, G.H., Jr. et al. "Results of treatment of carcinoma of the breast by local excision." *Surgery, Gynecology and Obstetrics* 132:780-2, 1971.

Dennis, C.R., et al. "Analysis of survival and recurrence vs. patient and doctor delay in treatment of breast cancer." *Cancer* 35:714-20, March, 1975.

"Earlier breast cancer detection told." Article in the *Los Angeles Times*, October 14, 1975.

Egan, R.L. *Mammography.* 2nd ed. Springfield, Ill.: Charles C. Thomas, 1972.

——— "Mammography, xeroradiography, and thermography." *Clinical Obstetrics and Gynecology* 18:197-209, June, 1975.

Ervin, C.V., Jr. "Psychologic adjustment to mastectomy." *Medical Aspects of Human Sexuality* 7:42+, 1973.

Fisher, B. "The surgical dilemma in the primary therapy of invasive breast cancer: a critical appraisal." *Current Problems in Surgery,* pp. 3-53, October, 1970.

Fisher, B., et al. "Postoperative radiotherapy in the treatment of breast cancer: results of the NSABP clinical trial." *Annals of Surgery* 172:711-32, 1970.

——— "Ten year follow-up results of patients with carcinoma of the breast in a cooperative clinical trial evaluating surgical adjuvant chemotherapy." *Surgery, Gynecology, and Obstetrics* 140:528-34, April, 1975.

Fisher, S. "Motivation for patient delay." *Archives of General Psychiatry* (Chicago) 16:676-8, June, 1967.

Fishman, J.R., et al. "Influence of thyroid hormone on estrogen metabolism in man." *Journal of Clinical Endocrinology* 22:389, 1962.

Fletcher, G.H. *Textbook of radiotherapy.* Philadelphia: Lea and Febiger, 1966.

Goldfarb, C., et al. "Psychophysiologic aspects of malignancy." *American Journal of Psychiatry* 123:1545-52, June, 1967.

Greer, S. "Psychological aspects: delay in the treatment of breast cancer." *Proceedings of the Royal Society of Medicine* 67:470-3, June, 1974.

Harrell, H.C. "To lose a breast." *American Journal of Nursing* 72:676-7, April, 1972.

Henderson, J., et al. "A psychiatric investigation of the delay factor in patient to doctor presentation in cancer." *Journal of Psychosomatic Research* 3:27, 1958.

Hoffman, V. "Cancer detection technique debated." Article in *Orange Coast Daily Pilot*, November 17, 1975.

Jick, H. "Reserpine and breast cancer: a perspective." *Journal of the American Medical Association* 233:896-7, August 25, 1975.

Kaae, S., and Johansen, H. "Breast cancer; five year results: two random series of simple mastectomy with postoperative irradiation versus extended radical mastectomy." *American Journal of Roentgenology, Radium Therapy, and Nuclear Medicine* 87:82-8, 1962.

Kushner, R. *Breast cancer: a personal history and an investigative report.* New York: Harcourt Brace Jovanovich, 1975.

Lasser T., and Clarke, W.K. *Reach to recovery.* New York: Simon and Schuster, 1972.

Lee, E.C.G., et al. "Proceedings: emotional distress in patients attending a breast clinic." *British Journal of Surgery* 62:162, February, 1975.

Leger, J.L., et al. "Report of the 'ad hoc' committee on mammography." *Journal of the Canadian Association of Radiologists* 25:3-21, March, 1974.

Leis, H.P. *Diagnosis and treatment of breast lesions.* Flushing, N.Y.: Medical Examination Publishing Co., 1970.

Leshan, L., and Gassman, M. "Some observations on psychotherapy with patients with neoplastic disease." *American Journal of Psychotherapy* 12:723-34, 1958.

Lobsenz, N.M. "What will our marriage be like now? Adjusting to a mastectomy." *McCalls* 100:55+, August, 1973.

"Lower radiation dose perfected." Article in *Orange Coast Daily Pilot*, November 6, 1975.

McCorkle, M.R. "Coping with physical symptoms in metastatic breast cancer." *American Journal of Nursing* 73:1034-8, June, 1973.

MacMahon, B., et al. "Etiology of human breast cancer: a review." *Journal of the National Cancer Institute* 50:21-42, January, 1973.

Medicine show, The; consumer union's practical guide to some everyday health problems and health products. Mt. Vernon, N.Y.: Consumers Union, 1974.

Meyers, T.J. "The psychologic effects of gynecic surgery." *Pacific Medicine and Surgery* 73:429-32, November and December, 1965.

Miller, S. H., et al. "Breast reconstruction after radical mastectomy." *American Family Physician* 11:97-101, May 1975.

Moss, W.T., and Bond, W.N. *Therapeutic radiology; rationale, technique, results.* 3rd ed. St. Louis: Mosby, 1969.

Nance, F. C. "Breast examination: differential diagnosis of breast nodules." *Clinical Obstetrics and Gynecology* 18:187-95, June, 1975.

Nelson, H. "Radioactive implants called effective in fighting cancer." Article in the *Los Angeles Times*, November 13, 1975.

Nelson, J. L. et al. "Epidemiology and treatment of breast cancer." *Clinical Obstetrics and Gynecology* 18:211-8, June, 1975.

O'Donnell, W.E. "Bad doctors—how can you spot them?" *Woman's Day* pp. 50+, October, 1975.

Owen, M.L. "Special care for the patient who has a breast biopsy or mastectomy." *Nursing Clinics of North America* 7:373-82, June, 1972.

Pangman, W.J., 2nd. "Breast trauma—surgical and psychic. Its repair and prevention." *Journal of the International College of Surgeons* 44:515-22, November, 1965.

Papaioannou, A.N. *The etiology of human breast cancer. Endocrine, genetic, viral, immunologic, and other considerations.* New York: Springer-Verlag, 1974.

Paterson, K. "After breast surgery." *Parents Magazine* 50:46+, January, 1975.

Peters, M.V. "Wedge resection and irradiation: an effective treatment in early breast cancer." *Journal of the American Medical Association* 200:144-5, 1967.

Reznikoff, M. "Psychological factors in breast cancer." *Psychosomatic Medicine* 17:96-108, 1955.

Rothenberg, R.E. *The complete book of breast care.* New York: Crown, 1975.

Snyderman, R.K., ed. *Symposium on neoplastic and reconstructive problems of the female breast,* volume 7. St. Louis: Mosby, 1973.

Strax, P. *Early detection; breast cancer is curable.* New York: Harper and Row, 1974.

Sutherland, A. "Psychological impact of cancer surgery." *Public Health Reports* 67:1139-43, 1952.

Sutherland, A., and Ohrbach, C. "Psychological impact of cancer and cancer surgery: II. Depressive reactions associated with surgery for cancer." *Cancer* 6:958, 1953.

Tarlau, M, and Smallheiser, I. "Personality patterns in patients with malignant tumors of the breast and cervix." *Psychosomatic Medicine* 13:117-21, 1951.

Thiessen, E.U. "Breast self-examination in proper perspective." *Cancer* 28:1537-45, December, 1971.

Titchener, J.L., and Levine, M. *Surgery as a human experience: the psychodynamics of surgical practice.* New York: Oxford University Press, 1960.

Titchener, J., et al. "The problem of delay in seeking surgical care." *Journal of the American Medical Association* 160:1187, 1956.

Vakil, D.V., et al. "Etiology of breast cancer. I. Genetic aspects." *Canadian Medical Association Journal* 109:29-32, July 7, 1973.

Vakil, D.V., et al. "Etiology of breast cancer. II. Epidemiological aspects." *Canadian Medical Association Journal* 109:201-6, August 4, 1973.

Watson, T.A. "Can survival be increased by postoperative irradiation following radical mastectomy?" *Journal of the American Medical Association* 200:136+7, 1967.

Weber, E., and Hellman, S. "Radiation as primary treatment for local control of breast carcinoma: a progress report." *Journal of the American Medical Association* 234:608-11, November 10, 1975.

Wheeler, J.I., Jr. and Caldwell, B.M. "Psychological evaluation of women with cancer of the breast and of the cervix." *Psychosomatic Medicine* 17:256-68, 1955.

Wise, L., et al. "Local excision and irradiation: an alternative method for treatment of early mammary cancer." *Annals of Surgery* 174:392-401, 1971.

Wolfe, J.N. *Xeroradiography of the breast.* Springfield, Ill.: Charles C. Thomas, 1972.

Woodward, K.L. "The cures doctors can't explain." *McCalls* 102:87+, April, 1975.

Zippin, C., et al. "Identification of high risk groups in breast cancer." *Cancer* 28:1381-7, December, 1971.

INDEX

Adrenal steroids,
level of, 35, 36
production of, 33, 40
Adrenalectomy,
performance of, 116
Age factor,
statistics on, 32
Anesthesia,
administering of, 98
type of, 96
Antibody,
amount of, 34, 35
Antidepressants,
as a cause factor, 39

Antigen,
amount of, 34, 35
Appointments,
for medical care, 65,
66, 67
American Cancer
Society, 65, 66
Anxiety,
following surgery, 122
Apprehension,
following surgery, 122
Arteriosclerosis, 37